# TEAL on WHEELS: Ovarian Cancer Awareness Tour

Coos Bay, Oregon to Swan's Island, Maine

August 28 - October 5, 2019

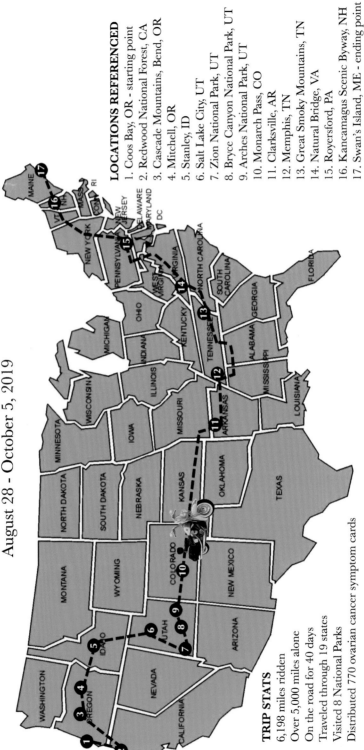

**LOCATIONS REFERENCED**

1. Coos Bay, OR - starting point
2. Redwood National Forest, CA
3. Cascade Mountains, Bend, OR
4. Mitchell, OR
5. Stanley, ID
6. Salt Lake City, UT
7. Zion National Park, UT
8. Bryce Canyon National Park, UT
9. Arches National Park, UT
10. Monarch Pass, CO
11. Clarksville, AR
12. Memphis, TN
13. Great Smoky Mountains, TN
14. Natural Bridge, VA
15. Royersford, PA
16. Kancamagus Scenic Byway, NH
17. Swan's Island, ME - ending point

**TRIP STATS**

6,198 miles ridden
Over 5,000 miles alone
On the road for 40 days
Traveled through 19 states
Visited 8 National Parks
Distributed 770 ovarian cancer symptom cards

# FINDING COURAGE

*Navigating Cancer on my Harley*

# FINDING COURAGE

# COURAGE

*Navigating Cancer on my Harley*

## DONNA WIEGLE

# FINDING COURAGE:
## Navigating Cancer on my Harley

Copyright © 2021 by Donna Wiegle

### SECOND EDITION

ISBN: 978-0-578-88476-9

Printed in the United States of America

Published by:
Donna Wiegle
PO Box 303
Swan's Island, ME 04685
www.tealonwheels.org
donna@tealonwheels.org

*A portion of the proceeds from this book will go to support Turning the Tide Ovarian Cancer Retreat, Inc.*

*To Charlie,*
*thank you for always believing in me.*

**Above all,**
**be the heroine of your life,**
**not the victim.**

*Nora  Ephron*

# Contents

# Chapter 1

# CLIMBING A MOUNTAIN

**As I sat on my motorcycle** at the base of the Rocky Mountains, winds howled all around me. I thought to myself, "What the hell am I doing here?" Crossing the Continental Divide was supposed to be one of the highlights of my trip, but instead I had arrived at the bottom of the majestic Rocky Mountains and couldn't make myself go any further. I shut the engine off, put my kickstand down, and sat there on the side of the road, contemplating my next move. Trucks and cars, heading east toward Monarch Pass, were passing me and all I could do was sit by the side of the road, all alone, consumed by fear.

Months earlier, at my home on Swan's Island, Maine, I was excited as I began planning my cross country trip. I would ride my 2016 teal and white Harley-Davidson motorcycle across the United States, starting on the West Coast and ride east until I got back home to Maine. I knew I would have to cross the Rocky Mountains and I looked forward to the challenge. I had searched the map of Colorado from north to south. Crossing the Rockies in September might present a slight chance of encountering snow while riding my motorcycle through a high mountain pass. As I scoured the map, I looked for a lower pass to travel up and over the Rocky Mountains hoping to avoid any bad weather. Route 50 East crossed over the mountains at Monarch Pass, elevation 11,312 feet. I could stay the night before in nearby Gunnison, Colorado, elevation 7,703 feet. It would be a short ride, less than 50 miles, from Gunnison to Monarch Pass.

My plan seemed like a good idea, but when I woke up in Gunnison on September 10, 2019, the temperature was 37 degrees—too cold for me to start riding and certainly too cold to climb up a mountain pass to 11,312 feet. I would have to kill some time waiting for the temperature to warm up a bit. I took off on my bike before breakfast and headed to a local car wash to give my motorcycle a bath. When I got back to the hotel, I headed to the lobby area to get some breakfast. I met a couple of bikers who were also killing time, hoping for a warmer start to their ride. They were heading to Monarch Pass that morning as well. We enjoyed chatting over breakfast about our unique mo-torcycle adventures—where we had started and where we were going. The men expressed surprise that a woman rider was out on the road all alone attempting such a long ride.

We met up again later in the parking lot outside the ho-tel as we were packing up our bikes for the day. I rolled out of the parking lot first and onto Route 50 traveling east. As soon as I left the protection of the buildings along Gunnison's main street and headed out of town, I was hit by a wall of wind that was whipping across the open space. Not just any wind, but the kind of wind that swirls around, not necessarily coming from one direction, but seemingly coming from all directions. On a motorcycle, this is not a comfortable situation. I am not a fan of riding in big wind and today was going to test me. The wind was 30-40 mph and gusting. I was forced to slow my speed and it took a great deal of concentration to keep the bike under control. The bike was being pushed from one side of the lane to the other. It was not going to be a fun day of riding—today was going to feel more like work.

About 20 miles into the ride, I could see two motorcycles off in the distance in my rearview mirror. I wondered if they were the guys I had met over breakfast. With each passing mile, the bikes grew bigger in my mirror. Eventually they got close enough for me to recognize them. It was the bikers from the hotel. They had steadily been gaining on me. When they finally caught up, I waved them around. I didn't want to slow them down. They gave me a hearty wave as they roared by.

I could see the Rocky Mountains up ahead. The closer I got, the bigger the mountains loomed. The wind had not subsided at all, and if anything, it seemed stronger. I stopped at a gas station just before I would be starting my climb up Monarch Pass. I filled up my bike's five gallon gas tank. My bike averaged around 50 miles per gallon, so I could ride about 250 miles on a tank. When I finished pumping my gas, a pickup truck that had just come across the pass from the east heading westward, pulled up to the pump opposite me. The driver, an elderly man with white zinc oxide coating his nose, got out to pump his gas. He was wearing a T-shirt sporting a Christian Motorcyclists Association logo on the front. His wife got out of the passenger side of the truck. I asked them if it was windy at the top of the pass. The wife responded that it was not. Her husband quickly corrected her citing that they had just come across the pass in their truck with the windows rolled up and pointed out to her that I would be going up on a motorcycle. He said, "Yes, it's very windy up there." I figured he knew something about riding by the shirt he was wearing. I shared with them my nervousness about climbing up the mountain. The wife, wearing a pink sweatshirt with an image of Jesus with a crown of thorns on the front, offered to say a prayer for me. Even though I am not religious, I gladly accepted her offer of prayer. This was only one of the many times on my trip that I would encounter someone who wanted to pray for me. She quickly finished praying and I was on my way.

I didn't travel far, just out of the gas station parking lot and across a small bridge, less than a mile. I pulled my bike to the side of the road and shut off the engine. This is where my fear took hold. I took my cell phone out of the pocket of my leather jacket. I was going to call Charlie, my husband. He was on the other side of the country in Maine, but I just wanted to hear his voice. Luckily, I had no cell phone signal. I say "luckily" because after almost 30 years of marriage, I know exactly what he would have said if I had been able to reach him. He would say, "I'm 2,500 miles away. What do you think I can do from here to help you? You just need to figure it out for yourself." Being married to Charlie has taught me to be independent. He would help me if I needed help, but he also wanted me to be able to solve problems on my own. I could hear his voice in my head and he was right—I just needed to figure it out for myself. I ran through my options. I could turn back and ride down to Arizona or New Mexico to get across the country, but that would mean hundreds and hundreds of extra miles and several days of additional riding, all because I was facing a challenge that frightened me. Or, I could just start the engine on my bike, shift it into gear, twist the throttle, and conquer this mountain. I chose the latter.

Life is full of tough choices, scary situations, unknowns—what you do during those times says a lot about who you are as a person. Are you a wimp, afraid of your own shadow? Or are you a warrior, ready to fight? Most of us fall somewhere in between the two extremes. On this day, I needed to be courageous. I dug down deep, found my courage, fired up the engine of my Harley, and forged up that mountain pass. It was windy, it was cold, and it was intimidating, but it was also beautiful, amazing, and inspiring. I stopped at several roadside pulloffs to take in the view and snap a few pictures. By the time I reached the summit at 11,312 feet, there was snow, not in the roadway, but on some distant mountain tops. It was cold at the summit and the wind at the top was probably gusting to 50 mph. I did not seem to mind it though. The hardest part of the ride was behind me now. Going down would be a piece of cake. I had such a feeling of accomplishment when I reached the summit. There was a parking lot with a small gift shop and cafe that I stopped at for a few minutes. In hindsight, it was

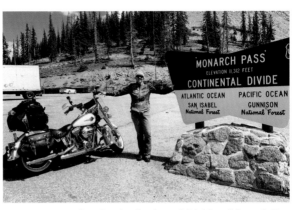

*Crossing the Continental Divide at Monarch Pass*

not as scary as I had built it up to be in my mind. As I stood at the top of the summit, I realized that anything is possible if you want it bad enough.

Climbing up Monarch Pass had a lot of similarities to how I felt in the spring of 2016, three years earlier, when I received a diagnosis of advanced stage ovarian cancer. Both were unfamiliar situations and both required courage to navigate. At that time, I had been working in the medical field for many years running a small health center on the island where I lived. I had enough experience to know the odds of me beating the cancer were not good. I had to accept my cancer diagnosis and learn to live with the side effects of the treatments that I would need to stay alive. After my first chemotherapy infusion, I was very sick. I remember saying to Charlie, "This is too hard. I don't want to live like this."

Getting through chemo had been a hellish nightmare. The treatment that followed the chemotherapy for the next few years wasn't any easier. My cancer had continued to grow. I was scheduled for surgery to remove a tumor in my chest as soon as I returned home from my cross country motorcycle ride in October 2019. My ovarian cancer had spread out of the pelvic/ abdominal area. The distant spread to my chest resulted in me being reclassified from stage IIIB to stage IV. In order to make the cross country ride on my timeframe, I had negotiated with my thoracic oncology surgeon, Dr. Gary Hochheiser. He wanted me to have the surgery in June, after a biopsy confirmed the tumor in my chest was indeed a spread of my ovarian cancer. My ride was planned to start in late August. I told him about my upcoming motorcycle trip and said I couldn't have the surgery until I got back. He assured me that I would be completely recovered by the time I was due to leave for my trip. I countered with, "What if something goes wrong? I'd have to call the trip off." At that point, my ride was the most important thing to me, and I was not going to let my cancer stop me. In the end, we agreed that I would have the surgery as soon as I returned home.

For me the ride across the country represented my last big hurrah. I didn't know how much longer I was going to live. I had decided to combine my love of riding with my longing to see the country by taking a solo motorcycle journey. I would start on the West Coast and ride home, all the way to the East Coast—from the Pacific Ocean to the Atlantic Ocean. My health had been steadily declining since my diagnosis. I didn't know if I could complete the trip, but I knew that I needed to at least start it. With each mile I rode, I felt more empowered.

# *Chapter 2*

# GETTING A DIAGNOSIS

**It was September 2013** and I lay on the bed shaking uncontrollably. I knew something was really wrong. I managed to get my cell phone and called Charlie to come home from work.  At the time, he was an EMT and I knew he could get me the medical help I needed. He hurried home from work to find me lying on the bed. He took one look at me and said, "You need to go to the hospital." Without hesitation, I agreed. I wanted to go.

I had been at Zumba, my exercise class, earlier that morning. I was having abdominal pain and did not feel well. I tried to convince myself that perhaps I had overdone it working in my garden the day before, or that I had lifted something too heavy and pulled a muscle. I was convinced I could exercise the pain away. But I could not. I had to leave the class and go home. I was a physically fit woman, age 53 at the time. I drove myself home and got into the shower. When I got out of the shower, I started shaking uncontrollably. Something was definitely wrong.

I was transported by ambulance from my home on Swan's Island, an island located 6 miles off the coast of Maine, to Mount Desert Island Hospital, a 25 bed facility in Bar Harbor. I had lots of tests performed and I was beginning to feel better. I was discharged without a diagnosis, but asked to return in a couple of days to have some free floating fluid in my abdominal cavity removed. They called it "ascites fluid". The doctor wanted to know what was in the fluid—possibly white blood cells, bacteria, or maybe something else.

I returned to the hospital as instructed and was taken to the room where they perform ultrasounds. Clear glass jars were lined up on a table. The ultrasound tech gave me a funny look and said, "You're not what I was expecting." I asked what he meant by that. He said most patients who have fluid removed are larger than me with extended abdomens. He continued on saying because I was of average size, without an enlarged abdomen, it made sense to him that they were doing the paracentesis procedure, a fluid extraction, during an ultrasound. He explained that all of the organs in your abdominal cavity are fairly close together. In a patient of my size, the risk of puncturing one of the organs during a paracentesis was a possibility.

The tech began the ultrasound and told me the radiologist would be joining us shortly. He would be the one who would insert the needle into my abdominal cavity to drain the fluid. The glass jars on the table would be filled with the fluid and taken for analysis. After some time, the ultrasound tech excused himself and left the room. I thought he was going to get the radiologist. He returned alone. He explained to me that he was unable to find the pockets of ascites fluid that had been present just a few days earlier when I was in the emergency room. He pulled up the ultrasound images I had done when I presented at the ER. He showed me on his screen black areas from the earlier ultrasound and told me this was where the fluid was. He then switched to the current ultrasound which revealed no black areas of fluid. There was no ascites fluid to drain. The conclusion was that my body had reabsorbed it, so I was sent home.

But, there was something wrong with me. I just didn't know what it was. Over the next two and a half years, I would periodically have these episodes, that's what I called them. An episode would begin with some abdominal pain that would increase in intensity over the next four to twelve hours. The pain became quite severe. It would culminate with a sudden onset of severe sweating, intense heat coming from the core of my body, and the most horrendous vomiting you can imagine. I would throw up everything in my stomach, plus the nasty green bile. By the time the vomiting was over I was drenched in sweat lying on the bathroom floor. I felt like I had just run a marathon. I was completely wiped out. I literally could not get myself up off the bathroom floor. The vomiting lasted maybe five to ten minutes, but it felt like hours. Charlie would have to come and help me back into bed. Afterwards, the abdominal pain would subside. The next day I would feel weak and I was dehydrated, but in a day or two I was back to normal. This went on for more than two years with episodes becoming more frequent. At first, it was every couple of months, then every couple of weeks. During this time I saw numerous specialists, had a battery of tests performed, but nothing revealed any answers. The episodes continued. I did not go to the ER during this two year period because the episodes were all self-resolving. Living on an island presented many challenges when trying to access emergency care. Charlie and I just dealt with them the best way we could, all the while knowing something serious must be going on. In April 2016, I had another one of my episodes. It was similar to all of the other episodes in many ways. The vomiting was over around 2am, but this time I did not get better. The pain did not resolve. When I was still suffering from incredible pain by 2pm, 12 hours later, I decided that I needed to go to the ER. An assessment and review of my symptoms, followed by a CT scan performed shortly after arriving in the ER revealed a bowel obstruction in my small intestine. It was a complete blockage. A nasogastric (NG) tube was placed up my nose, down my esophagus, and into my stomach. Having an NG tube placed is a horrible ordeal. Just pushing the large tube up my nose was bad enough, but then an overwhelming gag reflex came into play as the physician asked me to swallow so that the tube could be pushed down my throat. I was gagging the whole time. The experience was very traumatic. Over the years, I have been in the ER many times with bowel obstructions. I have only once agreed to another NG tube. I would rather suffer through the horrendous vomiting than have that tube inserted.

The job of the NG tube is to relieve the pressure on the top side of the blockage by removing all the contents in the stomach, including gastric juices and digested food. During a bowel obstruction you cannot eat or drink anything by mouth and must rely on IV fluids only. I once went six days with nothing by mouth, not even water. It was torture. The goal is for the NG tube to relieve the pressure on the blockage and that the IV fluids will keep you hydrated. IV pain medications are used to keep the patient comfortable until the obstruction resolves. Most bowel obstructions will resolve without surgery, but in April 2016, my obstruction would not resolve. It was the only time so far, of more than 20 bowel obstructions that I have suffered that I needed to have surgery.

On Sunday, April 17, 2016, after being at the hospital for several days, Dr. Charles Hendricks, my surgeon, came in to inform me that I needed surgery. I asked him if I should be transferred from the 25 bed rural hospital to a larger hospital in Bangor, Maine. He said he would make the arrangements if that was what I wanted. He told me I would be able to find a GI specialist in Bangor who was doing bowel resection surgeries all the time, but he added that my case was not typical. I had a belly full of pelvic radiation damage from treatment for cervical cancer 26 years earlier. He told me that I probably would not find a surgeon who had extensive experience with a patient with my complications. I asked him if he felt confident in doing the surgery and he said yes. In the days leading up to Sunday morning, Dr. Hendricks had made sure I was well informed as to what was happening each day and about the lack of progress in the small intestine. The longer we waited, the more there was a chance for part of the small intestine to die off and need to be surgically removed. Dr. Hendricks made sure I understood the situation. He would come to my room and unhook my NG tubing from the suction pump on the wall behind my bed and take me down to the nurses' station where he showed me the x-rays and lab results and discussed my situation. He treated me with great respect. I trusted him and I knew I would not find that bond with any other surgeon. I decided to stay in Bar Harbor at the familiar Mount Desert Island Hospital to have my surgery.

It was a beautiful Sunday morning. Dr. Hendricks told me he'd get the surgical team to come in on their day off to assist with the surgery. It wouldn't be long before they would be ready to go. I asked him to get the "A" team. I'm not sure, but being such a small hospital, maybe there is only one team, but I felt better asking for the "A" team. Dr. Hendricks left the room. I called Charlie and told him I would be having surgery and asked if he could come over to the hospital on the next ferry. He told me he'd be on his way and get there as soon as he could. I knew that meant I would not see him before I was wheeled into the operating room, but I hoped he would be there waiting for me when the surgery was over.

I rang the call bell for the nurse and asked her for a copy of Advanced Directives, a legal set of documents that I could fill out and express my end-of-life wishes as I would be unable to do so in the event that something went wrong during surgery. I did not want Charlie to have to make those decisions without having had time to discuss it with with me in advance. The nurse told me that Advanced Directives are something the social workers at the hospital handle and that there were no social workers there on Sunday. I told her I was familiar with the documents having helped patients on Swan's Island fill them out through my work at the island health center. I would just need two witnesses to sign once I had the document completed. I asked her to hurry as I didn't want Dr. Hendricks to know I was filling it out. I was afraid he might think it was a vote of no confidence in him, but that was not at all my intention. I was doing this for Charlie mostly, and for myself.

I knew from my conversation with Dr. Hendricks that I might end up with a colostomy bag. He explained that if they had to remove part of the small intestine that they would need two healthy ends to sew back together. Because of pelvic radiation treatment in 1990 for cervical cancer, my intestines were severely damaged and were a big part of the reason I was now having the repeated bowel obstructions. Between the pelvic radiation damage and adhesions from several abdominal surgeries over the years, my insides presented a very challenging situation. Oh how I dreaded hearing the words "colostomy bag". I told Dr. Hendricks I didn't think I could continue day after day in the hospital on morphine and IV fluids and I needed this to be resolved no matter what it took. I wanted to get back home and on with my life.

The surgery was successful. The bowel obstruction was cleared and I didn't end up with a bag. Dr. Hendricks told me that he found a couple of nodules on the outside of my small intestine and had sent them away for pathology. He didn't think they were going to turn out to be anything serious, but he said they shouldn't have been there. I was not terribly worried—after all I had already had cancer once and what were the chances of a second cancer. I didn't give it a lot of thought and would just wait until he got the report back. After a few days of recovery time, I was able to go home. I was sore and tired, but happy to be able to start eating again. I would have to change what I ate to try and prevent future bowel obstructions. I was instructed to eat a low fiber diet, which meant no vegetables, no fruit, no beans, nuts or seeds. It was not a very healthy diet, but it was thought that less bulk would reduce the number of bowel obstructions I was having.

About a week after I arrived back home from my hospital stay, I got a call from Dr. Hendricks. He said the pathology report concluded that the nodules were ovarian cancer. My heart sank when I heard those words. I'd been through this before when I was diagnosed with cervical cancer. In 1990, I had a hysterectomy, leaving the ovaries behind so I wouldn't go into menopause at age 30. At that time, the cancer had spread to my lymph nodes and I had 49 of them removed. I chose the most aggressive treatment at the time. My surgery was followed with 6 weeks of pelvic radiation to kill any stray cancer cells that may have remained. I had no idea what this new diagnosis of ovarian cancer would mean for me as far as treatment. I would need to see a specialist, a gynecological oncologist, to find out. Little did I know that my cervical cancer treatment in 1990 would be like a walk in the park compared to what would lie ahead for me this time.

## Chapter 3

# HOW MAY I HELP YOU

**We arrived early at Dana Farber Cancer Institute** in Boston, Massachusetts on a bright, sunny morning in early June 2016. Charlie and I had traveled there to get a second opinion about my cancer treatment options before making a final decision about starting chemotherapy at Mount Desert Island Hospital in Bar Harbor. Before heading to Boston, I'd had a consult with Dr. Laurie Small, a specialist in Gynecologic Oncology in southern Maine, and with Dr. Philip Brooks, an Oncologist at Cancer Care of Maine. Charlie and I wanted to be sure we understood all our options before making our final decision. At Dana Farber, I would be meeting with Dr. Alexi Wright, a medical oncologist, and Dr. Michael Muto, a surgical oncologist.

We had traveled to Boston, about 300 miles away from our home in Maine, the day before our appointments. Lucky for us, we had friends, Carolyn and Bill, who offered us their brownstone as a place to stay for the two nights we would be in Boston. Our friends told us to leave our car parked at the brownstone and take the T, the Massachusetts Bay Transportation Authority's transit system. We were a bit hesitant to follow their instructions, but on the morning of my appointments we made our way to one of the stations and got on the T. We hoped we were going in the right direction to get us to Dana Farber. Back in Maine we would have just asked someone for directions, but here in Boston every commuter was wearing earbuds and looking down as if they were intentionally trying not to make eye contact with anybody. I kept hoping for someone to look my way. Finally, I caught the eye of a young man and asked him for help. He showed us on the transit station map, on the wall of the railcar, where to get off. He further explained which direction we would need to go, on foot, to get to Dana Farber. It was a bit of a trek from the T station, up a long, windy hill to get to Dana Farber, but we eventually made it to our destination.

Adjacent to the 14-story Yawkey Center for Cancer Care, which houses Dana Farber, were other high rise medical facilities. This area, a couple of city blocks, must be the center of all things medical in Boston—where the top doctors in their profession practice. We had come to the right place to get some answers, or at least reassurances that what we had learned back in Maine was the right course of action to treat my cancer.

We felt dwarfed by all the tall buildings as we made our way along the sidewalk to the Dana Farber entrance. Busy traffic was zooming by and the whirl of helicopters landing on hospital rooftops overhead nearly drowned out our conversation. I couldn't tell you what we were talking about at that point. My mind was racing, just like the cars going by. I was anxious about what I would learn that day about my cancer and my treatment plan.

We entered the building and moved through the beautifully appointed lobby to a set of marble steps leading to the reception area. Each riser of the stairway had letters of gold on it. I stopped and read the words—HOPE, COURAGE, DIGNITY. I was suddenly overcome by the magnitude of what was happening to me—happening to us. I turned around and started walking toward the door we had just come through. Where was I going? What was I thinking? Charlie stopped me and we sat down next to a baby grand piano by the entry. I started to cry and told him I had to get out of there. We went outside and spotted a small garden area across the street. We went over and sat on a bench in a grassy area underneath all the towering buildings. I felt overwhelmed. I knew I would not be in Boston if this cancer wasn't something serious. I had overcome surgery and pelvic radiation treatment 26 years earlier for cervical cancer, but I knew this time it was going to be different. I had little hope of surviving this cancer.

Eventually, we made our way back into Dana Farber. We didn't want to be late for our appointments. This time we walked up the marble steps and proceeded to begin our day at this prestigious cancer institute, ranked #1 in New England and #4 nation-wide in 2016. We realized how fortunate we were that when we met with Dr. Philip Brooks, an oncologist who practiced at Mount Desert Island Hospital, he suggested we go to Dana Farber for a second opinion. Dr. Brooks made it very clear that he wasn't disagreeing with Dr. Laurie Small, my GYN oncologist in southern Maine, but he thought a second opinion was in my best interest before starting treatment. I was convinced that whatever happened at Dana Farber that day would dictate my course of treatment.

At the reception desk we were instructed to take the elevator to another floor where we would register, hand over the CDs with imaging that we had brought with us, and wait to see Dr. Wright, then Dr. Muto. When we got to this area, an older woman, wearing a blue vest, with the words "How May I Help You" on the back approached us. I thought she must have been a Wal-Mart greeter, at Dana Farber on her lunch break for a medical appointment. It turned out that Dana Farber has their own greeters. One thing that is etched in my mind from that day is meeting Anne Tonachel, one of the Dana Farber greeters.

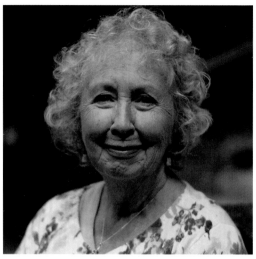

*Anne Tonachel*

Soft grey curls framed Anne's face. Her warm smile was welcoming. She asked, "Is this your first time at Dana Farber?" I wondered if our nervousness was showing. After all, we clearly were out of our comfort zone. All around us were patients and caregivers, doctors and nurses. The place was bustling with activity. Some of the patients were bald, or wearing scarves, or ill-fitting baseball caps, but underneath you could see they had no hair. Some were wearing face coverings and latex gloves indicating that their immune systems were shot—reduced from their cancer treatments. Would I look like that soon? I told Anne that we had come down to Boston from our home in Maine. I didn't notice at the time, but perhaps her eyes sparkled when I said, "Maine." She then politely said, "May I ask what type of cancer you have?" I replied, "Ovarian cancer." Again, I didn't see it, but I am sure Anne displayed a secret reaction to meeting an ovarian cancer patient from Maine. She explained to us how our day would unfold. We would see Dr. Wright first and that she would share her findings with Dr. Muto, who we would see second. Dr. Muto performed surgeries at Brigham and Women's Hospital, part of the Dana Farber complex. I was sure he would be the one doing my surgery. In Maine, Dr. Small had indicated I was not a candidate for surgery due to all of the pelvic radiation damage from my cervical cancer treatment 26 years earlier, but here I was in Boston. I was sure Dr. Muto would take me on as a high-risk surgical patient. After all, didn't I need to get rid of my ovaries? Unfortunately, I learned from Dr. Wright and Dr. Muto later that day that I was not a candidate for surgery. They both agreed with Dr. Small's treatment plan of weekly chemotherapy for 18 weeks and agreed that I would be able to have that treatment back home in Maine.

Back to Anne, she asked us to wait right where we were. She wanted to go and get something for me. She hurried off and quickly returned. She was holding a brochure for a retreat for women with ovarian cancer. Anne revealed that she was an ovarian cancer survivor herself. In 2012, Anne, along with fellow ovarian cancer patient, Robin Bray, began an ovarian cancer retreat for women in New England. Both Anne and Robin had attended an ovarian cancer retreat at Camp Mak-A-Dream in Montana and together they decided that ovarian cancer patients on the East Coast needed their own camp. The brochure was for the previous year's retreat, but Anne had crossed out the dates and put the 2016 dates. It would be in August. I was at Dana Farber in early June. I thanked Anne, but told her I would be in the middle of my cancer treatment in August and I didn't think I would be able to attend. I accepted the brochure and gave Anne one of my business cards. She stayed in touch with me through email over the next few months encouraging me to register for her Turning the Tide Ovarian Cancer Retreat held at Camp Kieve, a beautiful lakefront setting in mid-coast Maine, just 100 miles from my home. Anne said it would be fine to register and that I could cancel at the last minute depending on how I was doing with my chemo treatments. So I registered.

I didn't think much about the retreat as my health continued to decline throughout my weekly chemo treatments. I missed some weeks due to low white blood cell counts, low platelets, and low red blood cell counts. I charted my complete blood count numbers every week in a spreadsheet I had created. I could see how my counts would trend down with each week of treatment. Eventually, I'd have to have some sort of additional treatment to restore my white blood cell count or correct my anemia. My chemo consisted of two chemotherapy agents, Carboplatin (Carbo) and Paclitaxel (Taxol), given on week #1 of a cycle of three weeks. On weeks two and three I was only given the Taxol. Then the cycle started all over again. Three weeks made up a cycle and I was to have 6 cycles, or 18 straight weeks of chemo. Most patients undergoing chemotherapy go for treatment every three weeks, but because of the type of ovarian cancer that I was diagnosed with, low grade serous, I had chemo every week.

The retreat dates fell on a week where I should have had just the single agent Taxol for my treatment, but due to delays in treatment, it turned out that the retreat would start the day after I received one of my double agent treatments. The side effects on the weeks that I got the two chemo drugs together were always my worst. Weeks 2 and 3 of my cycle, when I only got the Taxol, were much easier for me. I had convinced myself that I wasn't going to be able to go to the retreat and had put it mostly out of my mind. I had been tracking my counts and was convinced that my blood counts would drop significantly the week of the retreat, but when I got to the infusion center that day and they drew my blood, my counts were okay, at least okay for a cancer patient. My red blood cell count and my hemoglobin were low, but not low enough to require corrective action. When my hemoglobin dropped, I experienced shortness of breath, sometimes very severe. That's when I would get an injection, a shot of Aranesp which is a treatment that is used to treat anemia caused by chemotherapy. I called Charlie and told him what my blood counts were and also told him that I wanted to go to the retreat the next day. He agreed and said, "Then you should go."

I also was under pressure by my two oncology nurses, Melanie and Joyce. Weeks earlier in talking about the retreat I told them there would be ziplining for anyone that wanted to do it and I wanted to do it. Melanie strongly encouraged me to go to the retreat. She said I had to do the ziplining. I didn't want to let her down.

The day after chemo was usually a pretty good day. At chemo, you get pumped full of steroids to prevent any allergic reaction to the chemo drugs. The steroid dose must be significant, because I always felt my best the day after chemo. As each successive day after chemo came along, I felt worse, until about day six when I started to feel a little better for a day or two, then back to chemo. It was a hard grind.

Anyway, the day following my double dose of chemo, I was pumped up on steroids and was able to get my suitcase packed. I was convinced I could drive the 100 miles to the camp where the retreat would take place and off I went. I arrived and was greeted by the lovely Anne Tonachel. Anne had stayed in touch with me through email since our initial meeting at Dana Farber and it was good to see her in person again.

My room assignment for the 5-day retreat would be up on the hillside, away from the main lodge where most of the activities and all of the meals would take place. I was excited to be there and to finally meet some other ovarian cancer patients. As soon as I got settled into my room I went down the hillside to the main lodge where all of the ladies were having a luxurious foot soak. What a great way to start the next five days of pampering, fellowship, and outdoor activities. It was immediately obvious to me as the women filed into the large room who was a returnee and who was a newbie like me. Those returning for the second, third, or fourth year of the retreat already had strong bonds built with the other women who had been there before. I felt kind of like odd man out, but that didn't last long. Everyone was very welcoming. I noticed that I was one of only two bald women at the retreat. Nola, the other bald woman, had been on her cancer journey for a long time, but was back doing another round of chemotherapy and had lost her hair again. The other women, who were done their treatment, or on drugs that didn't cause hair loss, had hair that spanned from very short hair that was just growing back or long hair. At first I thought Nola and I stuck out, but then I realized all of these women had been bald at some point in their treatment.

It felt good to be in the company of these cancer survivors, but little did I know then how hard it would become to be part of this cohort of amazing women.

There were many opportunities and activities that brought us together to share our stories and get to know each other better. The group numbered about 30 ovarian cancer survivors and about a dozen support volunteers and staff who provided us with wonderful meals, counseling, massages, facials, reiki, kayaking opportunities, music, and more. Each morning when we awoke, a bag of swag would be magically waiting outside the door of our rooms. The goodies might be edible, like chocolate bars, or things like boxes of tea, cards, lip gloss, a handmade pillowcase, candle—a wide variety of presents to start the day. Once you got showered and dressed and made your way down to the main lodge, more goodies awaited. A laundry line on the outside of the lodge was filled with beautiful handmade gifts attached to the line by clothespins. There were knitted hats, pairs of gloves, little cloth bags, shawls, neckwarmers—gifts all made with love from the many connections Anne Tonachel had fostered over the years. It felt good to feel so loved, and none of it would have been possible without Anne's inspiration and leadership. Robin Bray, the other co-founder of Turning the Tide, had passed away from ovarian cancer and now it was Anne making it all happen, along with many kindhearted volunteers that she recruited to help her.

Two very difficult things happened to me at the retreat that year. As each day of the retreat ticked by, I became sicker and sicker from my recent chemotherapy session. I could not eat and was having a hard time keeping up what little strength I had. I had a hard time staying hydrated. What little bit of nourishment I could get in me was rapidly leaving me when diarrhea, another chemo side effect, started. I was a shell of my former good health. I had always been athletic and competitive, but now I was a very sick woman, who couldn't carry her own suitcase to her room. I was physically and mentally drained.

The day for ziplining arrived and I was determined to do it no matter how weak I felt. I could not go back for chemo the following week and tell my nurses that I had chickened out. I didn't want to disappoint them, but more importantly I didn't want to disappoint myself. I still wanted to see myself as a whole person, physically fit and strong, even though I knew that was not the case. I had an image to uphold and so I was determined to go ziplining with the others. There were about ten of us who wanted to go ziplining that morning. We met at the main lodge after breakfast and a member of the Camp Kieve staff led us up the hill and into the woods. I was already experiencing shortness of breath by the time we stopped at the base of a towering telephone pole. We would have to climb the pole to get to the platform attached at the top. It was quite high up and that's where we would jump from, attached to the zipline overhead. We would fly through the woods, high up in the air, toward the end of the line several hundred yards away.

I didn't know how I would be able to do it. Several members of the camp staff helped us gear up. We had to wear a harness that would attach to the zipline and a helmet to protect our heads. I decided to go last. As I watched the others climb up the pole using the hand and foot holds, I thought to myself, I'll be able to do that. I'm not sure if any of the women were in treatment like me—mostly they looked healthy, as if their cancer was in the rearview mirror for them. They had long hair, indicating they were a long way past chemo. Some were younger than me, some older. They chatted and joked around and encouraged one another as each person's turn came around. As each jumped

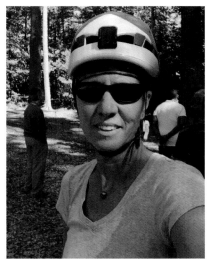

*Getting ready to go ziplining*

off the platform, they yelled out shrieks of joy and maybe a little fear. After all, this was the first time ziplining for many of us. By the time my turn came, the crowd at the base of the tall pole was small, just a couple of camp staff and a few onlookers who were there for support, but who were not going to participate in the activity. I began to climb up the pole. A young blonde woman, a camp staffer, was waiting for me to arrive at the platform. She would help me transition from the pole, over the edge and onto the platform. About halfway up, I lost all of my energy. I could barely breathe. I had completely underestimated the effect of my low hemoglobin on my oxygen level. Using all my muscles to climb the pole had depleted me of oxygen and thus my ability to breathe. I couldn't go up, but I couldn't come down either as I could not safely see the iron rungs sticking out of the pole beneath me. I was stuck, mid-way up, gasping for air. It was an awful feeling. I could feel my heart pounding in my chest. This was probably one of my top five times in my cancer journey where I became overwhelmed and just wanted to shout, "What the HELL is happening to me?" However, I didn't have the ability to shout anything. I felt paralyzed, hanging there on that pole. Thank goodness for the safety harness—if I fell I would not fall all the way to the ground, the harness would catch me.

Eventually I caught my breath and continued onward, up and to the edge of the platform. By the time I got there I was out of breath again. I said to the young woman waiting for me, "I am going to pass out." Everything was going black for me. She assisted me in getting up over the edge of the platform and sat me down. I stayed in that position for what seemed like forever. My helper was kind and patient and did not try to hurry me. The other women, the ones who went first, were waiting at the bottom of the line and could not see us. Eventually, someone walked back up the line to see what was taking me so long. I don't know how long I sat up there on that platform gasping for air. It seemed like an eternity, but finally I jumped off the platform and zoomed through the air, speeding toward the end of the zipline. I don't even think I enjoyed the ride, but I did it and for me that was the most important part.

When I got to the bottom and was able to get unhooked, the women waiting there gave me a bottle of water. They insisted on carrying my backpack and escorting me back to my room on the hillside. I am not good at asking for or accepting help, but these caring women weren't taking no for an answer. Together we made our way to my room. I lay down and thought about how awful that whole experience was for me. I thought about how far I had fallen from my former good health and about how much worse I would get by continuing my chemotherapy treatments. I wondered if I would ever get better again.

Later that night as the Turning the Tide ladies gathered for dinner, I joined them. As I looked around the tables at this amazing group of cancer survivors enjoying each other's company—laughing, smiling, sharing stories, and drinking wine, I thought to myself, they have all been where I am. They have all listened as a physician told them, 'you have cancer'. The many surgeries, chemotherapy and radiation treatments that this group of women had collectively endured was overwhelming, yet here they were enjoying life. At that moment, on the porch at Camp Kieve, surrounded by these beautiful and courageous women, I was given hope.

## Chapter 4

# TEAL on WHEELS - THE IDEA

**My husband Charlie and I** were planning a vacation to Arizona in January 2018. I wanted to rent a motorcycle and do some riding in the desert while we were out there. While I was out riding, I thought Charlie could just hang out with his good friend, Mike, who we were staying with outside of Phoenix. One day, Charlie came into my little home office when I had the Eagle Rider motorcycle rental page up on my computer screen. I was trying to decide which Harley-Davidson motorcycle model to rent for a week. I was leaning towards the Road King, a bike bigger and heavier than the bike I currently owned, a Softail Deluxe. Charlie said, "Get me one." I explained to him that he did not have enough riding experience. He had just gotten his motorcycle license only a couple years earlier and didn't even own a motorcycle. His only experience, besides the beginner motorcycle class he took, was riding my motorcycle probably less than 100 miles. I explained that there would be times when we would be riding on I-10, an eight lane highway. I continued on by saying traffic around Phoenix will be terrible in some places and I didn't want to have to worry about him as well as myself while I was riding. He was not taking no for an answer, so I made reservations for two Harley Road Kings for our upcoming vacation.

When we arrived in Phoenix, Mike picked us up at the airport. After a couple of leisurely days visiting with Mike and his wife, Kari, soaking up the Arizona sunshine, it was time to pick up our rental bikes. Mike drove us to the Eagle Rider rental location in Phoenix and dropped us off with our motorcycle gear. A customer service representative went over all the paperwork with us and went over the features of the two 2018 Road Kings. We picked out rental helmets, loaded our gear in the saddlebags, and fired up the bikes. By the time we got to the stop sign at the exit of the Eagle Rider parking lot, I knew I had made a mistake renting a bike this heavy. As soon as I applied the brakes, I could feel the weight of the bike underneath me coming to a stop. I quickly got my feet down. I thought about turning the bike around and going back to ask if they had a smaller model, but instead I pulled out onto the highway behind Charlie, and off we went.

Mike had told us about an interesting and scenic ride close to the rental location, where he promised there would not be a lot of traffic. It sounded like a great opportunity to get used to the bikes. We started off toward Apache Junction and to our ultimate destination, a lunch stop at Tortilla Flat. Tortilla Flat is an authentic remnant of an Old West town, nestled in the midst of the Tonto National Forest, in the Superstition Mountain Range. Tortilla Flat started out as a stagecoach stop in 1904. It sounded like an interesting destination. One thing I've learned over my years of riding, but didn't think about on that particular day, is to be careful taking advice about good places to ride from people who don't ride. Going somewhere in a car with four wheels under you is very different from riding on two wheels. The ride to and from

Tortilla Flat turned out to be one of those bad experiences. I'll give Mike the benefit of the doubt, he probably did not know that there was road construction going on when he told us to go there. The road down to Tortilla Flat was stripped of all asphalt and was down to bare dirt. To compli-cate matters more, it was a steep

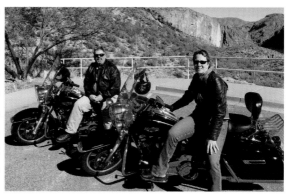

*Tortilla Recreation Site, Apache Junction, AZ*

downward incline, with sharp corners, and lots of one way traf-fic forcing us to stop frequently. The ride down was extremely nerve-wracking for me. I was glad when we finally arrived at the restaurant. I was relieved and knew I would never, ever, ride that road again. Over lunch I asked Charlie what he thought about the road heading out of Tortilla Flat going the opposite way than we had come. He quickly informed me that there was only one way out—the road we had just come down. My anxiety grew just thinking about stopping on the steep uphill inclines, holding our big, heavy bikes there, and then starting to go again, manag-ing the clutch and throttle simultaneously, and hoping not to roll backward down the hill, or do a burnout in the loose dirt. I was in the lead heading back up the road. It was slow going. At one point we caught up to a water truck that was spraying water on the dirt to keep the dust down. I could see the truck just ahead of me and thought, oh great, now we will be riding through mud. How much worse could this get. By the time we made it back to the paved roadway, I was so relieved to be able to open up the bike, shift through the gears, and feel the full power of this com-plex piece of machinery underneath me. We were still on a back road, but it was nicely paved. I was shifting through the gears and gaining speed when I saw a patrol car on the side of the Apache Trail Road. I eased off the throttle as I went blowing by the officer. I looked in my rearview mirror, but the car stayed parked. I smiled as I continued on my way.

By the end of the week when we returned the bikes, we had covered close to 1,000 miles and had enjoyed our time riding together. It was sunny and 70 degrees every day. Together, we had conquered Apache Trail to Tortilla Flat and managed to ride without incident on I-10 through eight lanes of super fast traffic. We made our way to Tombstone, Arizona, riding through the scenic valley of Sonoita, one of my favorite places to ride. The trip was a success. I enjoyed having Charlie with me on the road sharing the experience together. Most of my previous riding was solo, so the week had been a nice change for me. As a result of the trip, I decided that Charlie needed his own bike.

My mission that spring after returning from Arizona was to find a low mileage, used bike for Charlie, so we could continue riding together. I knew that I wanted to continue riding solo, but it would be fun to share some time on the roadway with Charlie, too.

My first stop to look for a bike for Charlie was North Country Harley-Davidson in Augusta, Maine. In 2010, I bought my first motorcycle there, a 2006 Sportster. My second bike came from Central Maine Harley-Davidson in Hermon, Maine, a 2014 Softail Deluxe. I was looking for something similar to my Softail Deluxe, a bike that not only Charlie would like, but one that I could comfortably ride, too. I explained to the salesman at North Country H-D what I was looking for and he showed me a 2016 teal and white Heritage Classic. My first and immediate reaction was, that's an ugly bike! I even went so far as to say, "No self respecting man would ever ride that bike." I thought the color combination was very feminine—even too much for me. Without finding any bikes there that interested me, I left the dealership.

Something about that unsightly teal and white bike kept finding its way into my thoughts. Teal was the color that represents ovarian cancer, just like pink represents breast cancer. Each type of cancer has a unique color representing it. I began thinking that if I could get that teal and white bike, that I could somehow use it to draw attention to ovarian cancer. I could ride it all over and spread a message of ovarian cancer awareness. There were several problems with my plan. First, I didn't need another motorcycle. I had a perfectly good motorcycle that I loved, but it was maroon. I had been on many adventures on that bike and I knew I was not ready to part with it—especially for something teal and white. The second flaw in my plan was money, or lack thereof. I worked, but my years-long journey with cancer consumed any extra money that was coming into our household. We were both self-employed, paying for our own health insurance. The premiums and high deductibles were crippling to our budget. There was no way I could make a case for buying another motorcycle just because it was the right color.

Month after month the idea nagged at me. If I could get that teal and white Harley, I could ride across the United States sharing my story and educating other women about the symptoms of ovarian cancer. I went back to North Country Harley-Davidson and asked to speak to the manager. I laid out my plan for him. I had even created a one-pager detailing what I intended to do with the bike. I asked him it they would lease the bike to me and I would return it at the end of the trip. He was not interested in any option other than a sale. I thought the bike was priced too high for its condition and mileage. The manager dropped the price, but it was still too much for me so I had to walk away. By now I was obsessed with the idea of using a motorcycle to spread awareness about ovarian cancer. I could not give up on my dream.

Around this time, I registered for a cancer conference, Stowe Weekend of Hope, held in Stowe, Vermont. I went to the conference, armed with several copies of my one-pager detailing my plan to ride a teal motorcycle across the country and raise awareness of ovarian cancer. I was staying at a rental house outside of town with a group of women from the Turning the Tide Ovarian Cancer Retreat. Anne Tonachel had arranged for the house and for us to all be together for the weekend. I shared my flyer, which included a picture of me sitting on that teal and white Harley at North Country's showroom. The ladies were excited about my plan and encouraged me to go for it, assuring me that I could do it. I had never done a trip of this magnitude. My longest trip had been 1,800 miles in a week. Crossing the country solo, as a stage IV ovarian cancer patient, would take courage, strength, and a lot of luck, if I was to succeed. One woman in particular, my friend Margaret, was the most supportive. The next afternoon, we went up the road to the von Trapp Brewery and Bierhall and had our first "business" meeting. I took notes as we discussed next steps and how we could make this happen. The first, and most important, next step was getting the right bike. Without this, there would be no cross country journey. At this point, I was all in.

Margaret, who lives in Massachusetts, continued to work with me, to support me, and to encourage me. She believed in me. Many, many phone calls and emails were exchanged over months of planning. We discussed fundraising. We knew we wanted to donate money to several ovarian cancer non-profits, including Turning the Tide Ovarian Cancer Retreat. We discussed how we would promote the project. Margaret came up with the name TEAL on WHEELS. I wasn't crazy about it, but I had no other idea for a name and so we just kept referring to it as TEAL on WHEELS and it took hold. I gave it a subtitle: Ovarian Cancer Awareness Tour. Things were moving along, but I still didn't have the bike yet. I began looking online to see if I could find one for sale.

Charlie's barber, Stacey, was a Harley rider and had bought all of her bikes at North Country HD. I stopped to see her to ask if she had any pull at the dealership. She didn't think she could help me. The bike was still there, two years after they first got it, but they still didn't seem willing to make a deal that I was comfortable with. I found the same exact bike for sale in New Jersey and one in Tennessee. The Tennessee bike, a 2016 model, was a good deal, priced right, and had all kinds of upgrades, GPS, heated seat, and only had a little over 1,000 miles. The seller was helpful in answering all my questions. I was curious about the many upgrades and why the bike had such low mileage. The seller told me that he became ill shortly after purchasing the bike and knew he would not be able to ride again so he was selling it. I looked into the cost of having the bike shipped to Maine. I was close to making him an offer when Charlie called me from the barbershop one day. He was there getting his haircut. He told me that Stacey had asked him if I was still looking for one of the teal and white Harley motorcycles. Charlie told her I was and that I

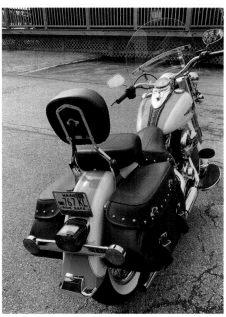

*Finally found the bike*

had found one in Tennessee. She told him there was one just outside of Ellsworth, in Lamoine, 25 miles from our home. I was elated. I put the Tennessee bike on hold and went to see the bike in Lamoine the next day. It was sitting at the edge of the road, in front of a motorcycle shop. It was in beautiful condition, had been garage kept, maintenance done, and only had 1,509 miles on it. A three year old bike with 1,509 miles—there had to be a story. I went in to talk to the shop owner. He told me a friend of his was selling the bike. The shop owner called the guy who was selling the bike, his buddy Mike. He told him I was there and that I was interested in the bike. We agreed that I would come back the next day, meet Mike, and take the bike for a test ride. After meeting Mike, I learned that he and his wife Sidney had bought the bike brand new after she passed her motorcycle class and had gotten her license. Sidney was a nurse, a mother of two teenagers, and just didn't have the time to ride, so they were selling it. The bike ran great on the test ride. There were a few obvious upgrades it would need to be road ready for a cross country trip. It would need to have stock handlebars put back on. The bike had been ordered with beach bars, lower handlebars, but I wanted the higher, little mini ape hangers, that were stock on this bike. I would also need to have engine guards and highway pegs put on. The upgrades could all be done after I owned the bike.

Mike and I agreed upon a price and I was off to the bank to take out a personal loan to purchase it. I really didn't want to enter into another motorcycle payment. I had only recently paid off my 2014 Harley, but with that paid off, I had the money to make payments on a new bike. I would be keeping my old bike and planned to sell the new bike when I returned from my trip in the fall. I didn't need two motorcycles at this point in my life.

I purchased the bike at the end of May 2019. That meant TEAL on WHEELS was now officially a go. There was so much work to be done. I planned to make my cross country ride in September, which was Ovarian Cancer Awareness Month. I thought it would be the perfect month, weather-wise, to make the trip. I knew I was not in good enough physical condition to ride out to the West Coast and back, so I planned to ship the bike west and ride home, completing my trip on the East Coast.

Margaret and I continued to work hard. Now that I had the bike, we could start the fundraising. We originally had three non-profits selected to raise money for and thought $10,000 each, so landed on a fundraising goal of $30,000. As we talked this over, we thought what if we got to $30,000 quickly—people will stop giving. We raised that amount to $50,000. I remember Charlie telling me that was too much, that we could never raise that amount, but we stayed firm on the $50,000. We set up a GoFundME page, but needed to be able to accept money from supporters who were not comfortable with donating online. We needed a fiscal sponsor. We did not have time to set up a 501c3 non-profit and did not want to go to all that work for a one-time event. I approached the Beth C. Wright Cancer Resource Center in Ellsworth, Maine. I knew Michael Reisman, the executive director, at the Center. I asked Michael if the Center could accept all the money that was donated both privately and through the

GoFundME page. He talked it over with his board of directors and they agreed to help me manage the money. Margaret volunteered to send out all of the donor acknowledgements for the GoFundME contributions. We were on our way.

Charlie was helping me with bike modifications. He installed my engine guards and highway pegs. Engine guards protect the bike if you drop it or if you have an accident. Highway pegs are attached to the engine guards, which are attached to the bike's frame under the windshield. Highway pegs give you the opportunity to get your feet off the floorboards and allow you to change foot position. For a ride of the distance I was planning, this was a must. We also found a way to convert the large, leather saddlebags to make them locking bags. The Heritage Classic does not have locking saddlebags and this was another necessity for a trip like I was planning. I bought a Garmin motorcycle GPS that hardwired to the battery, so we needed to get that set up and attach the loose wiring to the frame. The bike had a

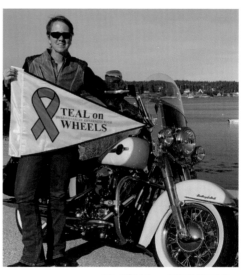

*My TEAL on WHEELS flag*

passenger seat where I could place an additional bag, but I also needed a luggage rack. I ordered one and Charlie installed that, too.

I felt like I needed a way to attract attention to my mission, so I designed and ordered a flag with a big teal cancer ribbon on it. It read: TEAL on WHEELS—Ovarian Cancer Awareness Tour. Charlie made a multi-piece flag pole made of plastic tubing that I could put on the bike when I wanted to display my flag. The short pieces of the flag holder easily fit in my saddle bag when I was not flying my flag.

Lots of motorcyclists wear leather vests adorned with the name of the riding club they belong to on the back of the vest. I bought a vest. I reached out to some of my motorcycle riding friends from the Widows Sons, a group of Free Masons who have a passion for riding. They wear big patches on the back of their vests and I knew they could tell me where to get a patch made

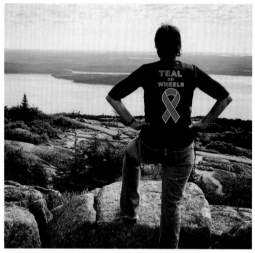

*My TEAL on WHEELS vest*

locally. I had an answer back in no time— LogoMotion in Brewer, Maine. I designed a patch on my computer. It had a large teal cancer ribbon and said Teal on Wheels. Next I needed to find somebody who could sew the patch onto the leather vest. I reached out again to my Widows Sons friends and got a name, Jan. I dropped the vest and the patch off at a bank in Milbridge, Maine, where Jan's daughter worked. I entered the bank with my vest in hand and Jan's daughter Tammy, said, "My mom just left. She's out in the parking lot." As luck would have it, Jan had just left the bank when I arrived and she was still in the parking lot. She said she would have the patch sewn on in a couple of days and would bring it back to the bank for me to pick up. I wanted to pay her upfront, but she would not accept any payment. She wanted to help me with my mission. This was just the first of many times that kind people donated their services to me to support my trip.

Everything was coming together. With each donation received toward the fundraising goal, my heart warmed. I felt the love of people near and far, those who knew me well, those who hardly knew me, and some who had never met me but still wanted to support TEAL on WHEELS. It was amazing.

As the day for my departure grew closer, my level of excitement rose. TEAL on WHEELS was actually happening. There was no turning back now. I had been interviewed by newspapers and had been interviewed on the bike for a health related story for a Portland TV news broadcast. I was already raising awareness about ovarian cancer before I even put the first mile of the trip on the bike.

*Chapter 5*

# BROTHERHOOD

**I bought my teal and white Harley** from Mike and his wife, Sidney. Mike is a member of the Low XII Riders Chapter of the Widows Sons, the International Masonic Riders Association. The Widows Sons members are a group of Master Masons who have banded together to enjoy motorcycle riding while emphasizing the tenets and principles of Freemasonry.

The Three Great Principles in Freemasonry are; **Brotherly Love**—Every true Freemason will show tolerance and respect for the opinions of others and behave with kindness and understanding to his fellow creatures. **Relief**—Freemasons are taught to practice charity and to care, not only for their own, but also for the community as a whole, both by charitable giving, and by voluntary efforts and works as individuals. **Truth**—Freemasons strive for truth, requiring high moral standards and aiming to achieve them in their own lives. Freemasons believe that these principles represent a way of achieving higher standards in life. The Widows Sons members that I have met through riding are shining examples of these principles.

There are Widows Sons chapters all over North America. Mike belongs to the Central Maine Chapter. Shortly after buying the motorcycle, Mike invited me to go on the 8th Annual Marvin Tarbox Memorial Ride with the Widows Sons. He explained that his chapter had voted to donate $300 to my Teal on Wheels cause and they wanted me to go on the ride with them. I had never participated in a group ride. I prefer solo riding, but Mike's invitation seemed like a good chance to try the group riding experience and to begin to raise awareness about my upcoming cross country ride. I wasn't sure how my message about ovarian cancer would be received by a group of motorcycle riding men, but I figured I had to start somewhere and this seemed like a good opportunity.

I had hoped to have my new motorcycle for the June ride, but it was still at the shop getting some modifications done. No worries, I washed up Little Ruby and got her ready for the ride. Little Ruby, a 2014 Harley-Davidson Softail Deluxe, was not all that little. She sported a 1690cc engine, one of Harley's 103 motors. We had been together since September of 2014, when I purchased the bike.

Mike invited Charlie to come on the ride as well. I confessed to Mike, who would be leading the day's ride, that I had never ridden on a group ride. He said I could ride in the front with him. He would lead and I would be right behind him. Charlie would not be riding with us, but would have to fend for himself somewhere back in the pack. Riding behind Mike felt more comfortable for me. I would only need to worry about one bike, the one directly in front of me.

The ride started at the Masonic Lodge in Ellsworth, Lygonia Lodge #40. When I arrived, there were already a bunch of motorcycles lined up in the parking lot. Guys and gals, dressed in motorcycle gear, most wearing leather vests with Widows Sons patches on the back, were socializing and greeting one another. I noticed some women accompanying the men had their own leather vests with Widows Sons Lady patches. I had entered a realm of the riding culture I was not familiar with, a brotherhood. They were not a gang, or a 1% club, but a group of men who came together to share a common love of riding and to represent the Masonic fraternity in a positive way. Not everyone on the ride was a Widows Sons member. There were other riders there that day, but the vast majority had a connection with the Masonic way of life.

I went inside the Lodge to register for the ride. The treasurer of the chapter was handling the registrations. He took my check and gave me a T-shirt made to commemorate the Annual Tarbox ride. I was asked to be near the front of the crowd of riders outside when the ride briefing began. I was told I would be presented with a check for the $300 donation at that time and would be invited to say a few words. This was not my normal type of gathering, and I grew nervous about what I would say. I wandered around for a while longer introducing myself to some of the bikers gathered both inside and outside the building.

As the time for our departure grew near, we were asked to gather near a newly erected flagpole in front of the building. The flagpole was the Eagle Scout project of Mike's son, Robert. We said the Pledge of Allegiance, and Robert was congratulated on the completion of his project, a proud moment for both him and his parents. The Widows Sons Low XII Riders Chapter President, Tom Spencer, presented a check to the local community college in Marvin Tarbox's name. Next, he invited me to come forward and presented me with a check for $300. Mike gave me an additional $245 in cash, half of the 50/50 raffle proceeds from tickets that were sold earlier that morning. Then, Tom invited me to say a few words. I explained that I was a stage IV ovarian cancer patient and that I was planning to ride the motorcycle that I had bought from Mike and Sidney on a solo trip across the country in September to raise awareness about ovarian cancer. I thanked the crowd for their generous contribution to my fund-

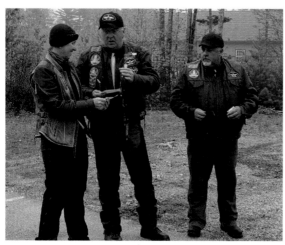

*Receiving the donations from Tom and Mike*

raising efforts citing that I hoped to raise $50,000 to donate to several ovarian cancer non-profits.

The ride briefing came next; what to do, where we were going, how to ride in staggered formation, hand signals, and blockers, and lastly, we were told to have a safe ride and enjoy the day. We saddled up and Mike and I pulled to the head of the pack. As we rolled out of the parking lot, I could hear the rumble of about 100 motorcycles following me. My ride to the Lodge that morning had been through some dense fog. The fog was now lifting and it was going to be a beautiful late spring day on the coast of Maine. We headed toward Mount Desert Island, where we would ride down Somes Sound and into Northeast Harbor. From there, we would loop back toward Acadia National Park and take a shortcut through the Park to Route 3 and back toward Ellsworth. As we made our way along the route, the riders behind me did their best to stay close. As we climbed up Dreamwood Hill leaving Bar Harbor, I looked back in my rearview mirror and saw an amazing sight. The bikes stayed in a tight formation up the hill and I could see all the way to the back of the pack. I had no idea where Charlie was, but I knew he was back there somewhere. We pulled into the Dysart's gas station off Route 3 just a few miles short of Ellsworth. I didn't need any gas, but many of the riders pulled their bikes up to the gas pumps and filled up. Some went inside for a bathroom break and others took advantage of the stop to smoke a cigarette. After about 15 minutes, we got on our way again. We turned right onto Myrick Street and then another right onto Route 1 East.

Our destination was the Masonic Lodge in Milbridge, where the members were preparing a lunch for us. Now that we were out of the Ellsworth and Bar Harbor traffic, Mike twisted his throttle and opened up his engine. We were running down Route 1 at a comfortable pace. The pack of bikes behind me seemed to grow smaller in my mirror. Mike slowed down several times and we could see they were gaining on us, but they never did close the gap before we got to the Pleiades Lodge #173 on Bridge Street in Milbridge. Eventually everyone arrived, parked, and the lunch and social time began.

Brent and Howard, two of the Pleiades Lodge members, presented me with a second check for $100. This would be the my first time meeting How-

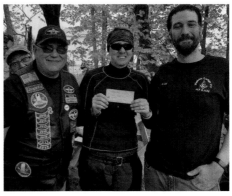

*Howard, me, and Brent at the Pleiades Lodge*

ard, but not my last. There was something special about him. He was funny and warm and seemed to be well liked by everyone. I could see why. Howard was a member of the Widows Sons Low XII Riders Chapter. We would become friends and he would be part of a group of riders that would accompany me on my very last day of Teal on Wheels.

I shared my story and gave out ovarian cancer symptom cards to a lot of people that day. At one point, a group of women, the ones wearing the leather vests with the "Lady" patches, approached me and presented me with a Low XII Riders Widows Sons "Lady" Medallion. It was a coin, two inches in diameter, with substantial weight to it. It was beautifully adorned on one side with the all-seeing Eye of Providence used to represent the omniscience of God, a common symbol used by the Masons. On the back side it was engraved, "Widows Sons Lady—Supporting our Masons". It also showed an outline of the state of Maine and a lady's slipper. On top of the slipper was a square and compass, another symbol used to represent the Masons. The coin was in a heavy duty plastic pouch for protection. The women told me that as long as I had this coin in my possession traveling across the country, Masons were obligated to help me if I needed it. It sounded kind of like a Masonic "AAA" coin. The coin stayed in my pocket the whole way across the country on my Teal on Wheels trip. It was comforting knowing it was there.

There was no organized ride back to Ellsworth. As things began to wind down, riders made their way to their bikes to head home. Charlie and I lingered to talk with more people. We had enjoyed the day, our first group ride, the comradery of the group, and the support given to me for my cause from people who didn't even know me. The last person I spoke with before we left for home was a boat builder from Milbridge. His name was Joe. Nearly everybody was gone at this point as Joe approached me and introduced himself. He handed me some dollar bills folded up in his hand. He wanted to make a donation in addition to what I had already received from the two Lodges. I put the money in the pocket of my leather chaps. We chatted some more about boats and Swan's Island. He knew some of the lobstermen from my island. We parted ways and I thought to myself, what a nice guy. It wasn't until Charlie and I got back down to the ferry terminal in Bass Harbor and had boarded the ferry that I reached down into the pocket of my chaps and pulled out the wad of money. I unrolled it. There were ten $20 bills! Joe, a man I had just met, gave me $200. I quickly asked Charlie if he had gotten Joe's last name. He had. Joe and Charlie parked next to one another when they arrived at the Lodge in Milbridge. They had had a quick conversation and exchanged names. I was relieved that I would be able to get an address so I could send Joe a thank you note. Since that day, Charlie and I have gone out to dinner with Joe and his wife, Victoria, and I have visited Joe at his boat shop in Milbridge numerous times when I ride in that direction in the summer. Joe invited us on another charitable ride later in the summer with his Widows Sons chapter, the Wayfarers. This time I was riding my teal and white Harley and proudly flying my Teal on Wheels flag.

Through Joe I have met more Widows Sons members and have become Facebook friends with many of them. I am astonished at the brotherhood, the bond that they share is so strong. I am proud to be part of the fringe group that respects the good work that the Widows Sons, Masons, and Shriners do. I watched as they completed a much needed renovation of a house for one of their brothers, and my friend, Howard, aka Chopstix. Howard was diagnosed with end stage liver cancer and lost his life in a few short months in November 2020. He had a dying wish. He shared with me one day, "I am laser focused on getting this house done for my wife Tracie before I die." Charlie and I stopped by Howard and Tracie's house one weekend on our bikes. There was a crew of Masons there working like crazy to get that house finished for Howard—to honor his dying wish. That was an incredible example of love for a brother.

*Chapter 6*

# DAY NUMBER ONE

**A cross country motorcycle adventure** sounds like a lot of
fun when you are lying in bed at night thinking about all the interesting and beautiful places you would want to visit. I recalled
scenic images I had seen in magazines and on the internet. I
consulted maps. Planning the route I would take was exciting.
A few years earlier, I'd completed a couple of solo motorcycle
trips to Canada to circumnavigate the Gaspé Peninsula and the
Cabot Trail. The longest of those two trips was 1,800 miles and I
was on the road for a week. I learned a lot about myself on those
trips and they certainly helped to broaden my knowledge about
long distance riding, but a trip across the United States would be
many more miles and would take a lot longer. I imagined I would
ride about 6,000 miles and be gone from home for a month. I
thought I could average about 200 miles a day, giving myself

plenty of time to meet people and share my message of ovarian cancer awareness. I also wanted to make sure I had some time to visit some of the scenic places along the way as I traveled across the country. I worried about my health—whether or not it would slow me down. I wasn't sure I was physically up to the challenge, but I was committed to going and committed to my mission.

I planned the trip for the month of September to coincide with Ovarian Cancer Awareness Month. All cancers have a color that represents them and a month designated as an awareness month specific to that type of cancer. I was pleased that Ovarian Cancer Awareness Month fell in September and not January or February, or some cold weather month. September seemed like the perfect month to ride across the country. Tornado season was over, summer was coming to an end, and winter was still months away—September would be perfect, at least that's what I thought.

As I studied maps of the country, I consulted Mapquest on my computer to figure out the mileage between the places I wanted to go. In the beginning, I thought I would map out the whole trip, plan where I would stay each night, and have an itinerary that I would follow to get me from the West Coast back home to the East Coast. I knew from the start that I couldn't ride from Maine to California and back again, so I chose to ride just one way—west to east. I didn't think I could physically endure a roundtrip adventure and I also didn't think I could be away from home for that long, even if my health remained stable.

I decided to ship my bike to the West Coast and ride east. I wanted to end my ride at home in Maine. I'm not sure how I came up with Oregon as the place to begin my ride, but a phone call to a Harley-Davidson dealer in Coos Bay ended with me knowing that it was the right place to start. I spoke with Karen, the owner of Highway 101 Harley-Davidson. When she told me that her dealership was the western-most Harley dealer in the continental United States, I immediately knew that I had found my starting point.

My next hurdle was finding an affordable way to get my

bike from Maine to Oregon. I did a search online to find a shipping company that would transport a motorcycle safely across the country. I found all kinds of companies willing to take my bike and my money. In the end, I chose the most expensive one. Prices for the one-way transport ranged from $600 to $1,200. I needed to ship my motorcycle fully loaded. I was taking a lot of gear on the trip and I wanted to ship it on the bike. I had packed 1,000 ovarian cancer symptoms cards in gallon size ziplock bags and stored them in my saddlebags, along with rain gear,

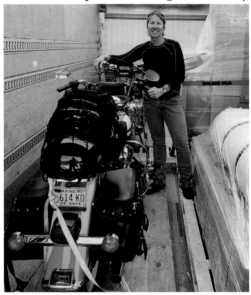

*Loaded and ready for transport to the West Coast*

tools, a first aid kit, flashlight, maps, extra gloves, neck warmer, hats, and so much more. The saddlebags were filled to capacity. Some of the transport companies told me I couldn't ship the bike packed, others said I could. The company selected, Federal Transport, would allow me to ship the bike with both saddlebags packed and an extra bag with all of my clothes attached to the passenger seat. I used a stretchy cargo net and attached my helmet on the luggage rack behind the passenger seat. I purchased extra insurance to fully cover the cost of the motorcycle and all its contents. I only wanted to take a small carry-on bag through the airport when I flew west. That bag would contain my good camera, a GPS, my iPad, my medications, and few other incidentals. It would be attached to my luggage rack once I started the trip. I would wear my motorcycle boots on the plane. I was charged extra for the motorcycle shipping for remote pickup and remote drop-off. Apparently, Maine and Oregon are not located on any major routes for shipping. The company agreed to pick up my bike in Ellsworth, about 25 miles from my home.

I was given a timeframe of four days, August 5-9, for the pickup, and told I would get a call the day before. Living on an island, connected to the mainland by a ferry, makes it a little challenging to be "on-call". I had to be ready to leave the island at any time and be in Ellsworth when the truck arrived to pick up my bike. I finally got the call and left the island the following day on my bike. It was a rather warm August day and I arrived at the designated meeting spot, the parking lot in front of the TJ Maxx. I arrived early and waited patiently for the truck to arrive. Eventually, I saw a large box truck approach. The driver pulled in and made his way to where I was parked. We decided to go out behind the store to load the bike. There were two men in the truck, the driver and his helper. When we got out behind the TJ Maxx building, they went right to work. First they inspected the bike looking for any scratches, dings, dents, or paint imperfections—it was all recorded down on their log. They opened the back of the truck and lowered the lift gate. I could see inside the truck and spotted another motorcycle sitting securely toward the front of the cargo area. I felt some relief. I could also see other items, not motorcycle related, that they were hauling. The boss of the operation, the driver, questioned me about shipping the bike with my gear onboard. I told him I was willing to take the chance of shipping with all my gear on the bike and that I had paid for extra insurance. I told the men about the purpose of my trip and that I was a stage IV ovarian cancer patient. After the bike was loaded onto a pallet and in the back of the truck, they used ratchet straps to securely fasten it down. I asked if I could get in the truck and look it all over. The boss said customers were not allowed inside the truck. I pleaded my case and he let me get in. I checked over all the straps and was satisfied that the bike would be fine for the long journey. I pulled out a cargo net and placed my helmet on the luggage rack and fastened it tightly. I said goodbye to my beautiful teal and white bike, which I had only had for about eight weeks at this point. I was hoping that when we were reunited at the end of the month on the

West Coast that everything I had packed on the bike would all be there.

My motorcycle arrived as planned and I picked it up at Highway 101 Harley-Davidson in Coos Bay three weeks later on the afternoon of August 27. I had flown from Portland, Maine, to Washington, DC, to San Francisco, CA, and onto North Bend, OR after getting an early morning start. I took a taxi from the North Bend airport to the Motel 6 where I was staying in Coos Bay, stashed my stuff in my room, and walked to the Harley dealer, about a mile away.

I programmed the address of the Harley dealership into an app on my phone and followed the directions to my destination. I was wearing my leather boots, jeans, T-shirt, and my leather vest with TEAL on WHEELS and a teal cancer ribbon embroidered on the back. I was geared up and ready to go. When I arrived, I approached the counter and stated my business—I was there to pick up my motorcycle. All of my communications involving the delivery to Coos Bay were with Karen. She was great on the phone every time we talked and was more than happy to accept my bike when it arrived on the West Coast. The young woman at the counter went in the back to get Karen. She came out and seemed glad to finally meet me, and I was glad to finally be standing in her dealership, ready to start my trip. Karen told me my bike had just arrived the day before. I was surprised since I had shipped it three weeks earlier, but nevertheless I was glad it was there. I was anxious to see the bike, check its condition, and to make sure all my gear was still safely aboard.

I asked Karen how much I owed her for taking delivery of the bike. She knew what my ride was all about. I had already given out three ovarian cancer symptom cards to her and two other women working at the dealership. I had given them my canned speech about ovarian cancer's symptoms and how difficult it is to get a diagnosis. Karen responded, "No charge. I am happy to be able to help you." She then instructed me to pick out any shirt in the store at no charge. I chose a long-sleeve T-shirt with a lighthouse on the back. It reminded me of home, the coast of Maine.

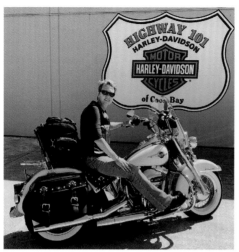

*Reunited with my bike at Highway 101 H-D*

The shirt wasn't really teal, but it was the closest to teal in the showroom, so I decided it was the right one.

Karen invited me behind the counter and led me down a long hallway. I spotted my bike up ahead. It was so good to lay eyes on it. A young service technician came out of the garage area. He had received the bike the day before and had gone over it with the transport driver. He asked me to look over the bike to make sure it was in the same condition as when it left Maine. A quick look satisfied me. The technician pushed the bike outside for me parking it in front of a big Highway 101 Harley-Davidson sign. Karen told me to hop on the bike and she'd take a picture of me before I rode off.

I was excited to take the bike for a ride. I would not be leaving Coos Bay until the next morning, but I wanted to take a spin to make sure everything was working properly. I put my helmet on and took off for a short ride. I had shipped the bike with the gas tank close to empty, so I pulled into the first gas station I saw and filled up the tank. I rode south on Highway 101 for a little while before turning around and heading back to the Motel 6. I parked the bike right outside of my ground floor room.

I was hungry and tired from the long day of travel. Karen had told me about Walt's Pourhouse, a pub that was a short walk away. I decided to go and get some grub and have a couple of beers to celebrate the start of the trip. It had been a lot of work to get to this point. I sat at the bar and engaged in conversation with another patron. Just as I was finishing a tasty burger and fries, Karen came through the door with her husband. She invited me to join them, but I was nearly done eating and I needed it to be an early night. I declined her invitation and thanked her again for all that she had done to help me get to the starting point of my journey. I was excited for the next morning to come so I could set off on what I imagined would be a trip of a lifetime!

I knew from all the endless hours of studying maps that the Redwood National Forest in California was about 140 miles south from Coos Bay, straight down Highway 101. I had always wanted to see the towering giants. On day number one, I would take Highway 101 South to California to see the redwoods. I didn't sleep well that night. I was far too excited for sleep. My body was still on East Coast time and I just wanted to get started. Each time I pulled the curtain back and looked out the window of my room, hoping for daylight, all I saw was darkness. I finally got out of bed, showered, dressed, and worked on packing the bike. It was still too dark to leave, but I could tell it was going to be a foggy start to my ride once the sun came up. No worries, I live in Maine where we have fog all the time. At the first light of dawn, I fired up the bike and headed out of town. The fog made for chilly riding. I stopped and put on warmer gloves and a polar fleece neck gaiter. It was not the kind of day I was hoping for to begin my ride, but my excitement outweighed all other factors and nothing else mattered.

The ride along the Pacific coast was amazing—ocean views and windy roads! The further south I went, the less fog I had. It was beginning to warm up a little. I pressed on enjoying every mile and dreaming about the things I would see on this trip and the people I would meet. I began to see magnificent trees along the edge of the road and eventually came to a sign announcing I had arrived at my destination—Redwood National and State Parks. I slowly entered the park area. As I continued on I became dwarfed by the towering redwoods. I made my way to a small parking area across from a meadow where elk were bedded down. Every space in the parking lot was full. I decided to pull my bike off the edge of the paved area near the last spot. No one would mind a motorcycle sitting there.

I had a job I needed to accomplish and the edge of the

parking lot worked just as well as any other location. I had received a vanity plate for my teal and white motorcycle compliments of my friend Steve, who runs a Facebook page called Motorcycle Riders of Maine. Steve was a big supporter of mine, and he insisted that I have a vanity plate and he wanted to pay for it. Steve would not take no for an answer. Steve is a unique character. If you crossed him on his Facebook page, he'd boot you out of the group, no questions asked. He had rules and you needed to follow them. I got along well with Steve, but many of my other riding friends have gotten the boot over the years. One of Steve's suggestions for my vanity motorcycle license plates was O-V-A-R-I-A-N—seven characters, the maximum allowable for a motorcycle plate. I couldn't imagine riding down the highway on a motorcycle with OVARIAN on the back. What would people think? I tried to picture a guy riding a motorcycle with TESTICLE on his plate. It would be too many characters, but you get where I am going with this. Steve and I finally agreed on TEAL—teal being the color that represents ovarian cancer. The vanity plate arrived in the mail after I had shipped the bike, so I brought it with me on the plane the day before and now I needed to install it.

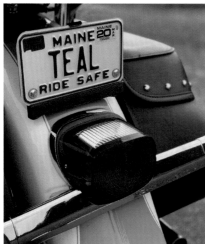

*TEAL vanity plate installed*

As I was crouched down at the back of the bike, removing my old license plate, a jacked up, extended cab, black pickup truck with a super loud exhaust system and tinted windows pulled up next to me. It had a Nebraska tag and a big CORNHUSKERS decal in the back window. It sat next to me, blowing exhaust and loudly idling for a considerable amount of time. I became rather annoyed by the smell and sound of the exhaust and looked up to see why it was just sitting there. It was waiting for a car to pull out of a parking space in the crowded lot. As soon as the car backed out, a small Subaru, coming from the other direction, sped into the parking space in front of the truck. The truck lurched forward with the horn blaring. The driver jumped out and a string of obscenities began pouring from his mouth. I looked around at this beautiful park I was in, at the serene meadow with the elk across the way, and thought to myself, what an asshole! The lady in the Subaru agreed to vacate the space. She was probably terrified! After the pickup truck pulled into the spot, two women got out of the back and headed toward the bathroom. The driver and another man got out of the front of the truck and were heading my way. I was still bent down behind my motorcycle and as they got closer to me I looked up and said, "Was that really necessary?" The driver started spewing one excuse after another about how the car stole his spot. I quietly responded, "I saw that, but you could have handled that better." He seemed to calm down a bit after I confronted him. His friend, who revealed that he was a motorcycle rider, asked me about my bike and if I had ridden all the way from Maine when he saw my tag. I explained to them that I was just starting a cross country trip to raise awareness about ovarian cancer. I gave them two ovarian symptom cards to give to their women who were still in the bathroom. They walked away. The women rejoined them and they all sat down at a nearby picnic table. I was finishing putting my new TEAL plate on the bike when the men came walking back toward me. One continued past me to their truck and the other one stopped to talk to me again. He handed me a one-hundred dollar bill and told me to put it toward my trip. I thanked him for his generosity and he walked back to the picnic table where the women were still sitting. The other man who had gone to the truck walked over and handed me some folded up bills which I put in the pocket of my leather chaps. He echoed the same sentiment about using it for my trip and walked away. He had given me two one hundred dollar bills. The two men, that I confronted about their bad behavior, gave me $300. I realized at that point that my story and my message of ovarian cancer awareness resonated with people—all kinds of people. This was going to be an interesting adventure.

## *Chapter 7*

# MEETING AL

**My friend Al is one of the most unique individuals** I have ever met. My first encounter with him was through social media and I immediately fell in love with his overwhelming sense of kindness, or goodness, or whatever it was that drew me to want to know more about him. Al saw the best in every situation. He was always positive. He was someone I wanted to meet.

When we met for the first and only time, it was 3,000 miles away from where we both started, me on Swan's Island, Maine and Al at his home in Weymouth, Massachusetts. Our paths converged in Oregon, of all places, on a bright sunny, summer day. Al knew I was traveling through Oregon on my Teal on Wheels ride and he was living near Portland so we planned to meet up and ride together.

Al is the kind of guy who would be willing to ride anywhere, no matter the distance, to meet up with a friend—even a friend he had not yet met. We agreed to meet in the Cascade Mountains, outside of Bend, Oregon. A guy I met at a bar, while having dinner the night before, told me I shouldn't leave Bend without riding this nearby area. Al offered to get an early morning start and ride several hours south from Portland to meet me at the beginning of the Cascade Lakes Scenic Byway, just outside of Bend. The scenic byway was a 66-mile roadway running through the rugged country of Deschutes and Klamath counties on the east side of the Cascade Mountain Range. I arrived at our agreed upon meeting place first and was waiting at the entrance to a small parking lot. The parking area offered a fantastic view of the snow covered Mount Bachelor, the highest point in the Cascade Mountain Range at 9,068 feet. I patiently waited for Al to arrive enjoying my early morning view of the mountains.

I was not waiting long when I saw Al making his approach. I flagged him down as he neared the area where I was parked. He made the turn into the lot and as he did I got my first glimpse of him, his motorcycle, and the trailer he was towing behind his bike. The image of rider and trailer was nothing like I had ever seen before in person. I've seen motorcyclists towing trailers before, but nothing like this rig. I knew Al had towed a trailer with him on his ride across the country, but I guess I didn't expect to see it trailing behind him when he pulled into the parking lot that morning. It was not your typical motorcycle trailer, but nothing about Al was typical. His bike, an older Honda VTX 1800, was covered with a couple of year's worth of bugs on the windshield and the fairing. It would have been nearly impossible to guess when he last washed it. But that was not the thing I noticed first about the bike. What caught my eye as Al pulled in and came to a stop was a skull, I'm guessing a deer, with an 8-point rack, mounted on the front of the bike. That wasn't all—the skull was wearing an old set of riding googles strapped to it over the empty eye sockets. The unusual nature of this motorcycle didn't stop there. It was sporting a vehicle tire on the back—a tire that looked like the size of one of my pickup truck tires. The rearview mirrors on the bike were attached to the handlebars by brackets that looked like the bony hands of a skeleton. Everything about the presentation was unique, just like Al.

As he got off his bike, I got my first head-to-toe look at this 26-year-old young man. His slender body was sporting skin-tight black jeans that were tucked into the combat boots he wore on his feet. On his top half, he was wearing a hand-woven, black and white striped, Mexican looking tunic and around his neck, a schmeg, a Middle Eastern tactical scarf. Tying the bottom and top of his outfit together, at his waist, he wore a belt made of shiny, pointy bullets—

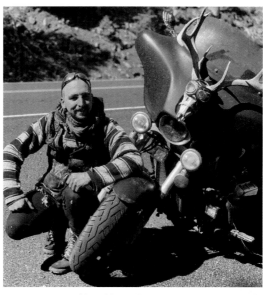

*Al and his uniquely adorned Honda VTX*

the kind I imagined would be used in a high-powered rifle. Dangling from the belt were several chains, the kind that might hold a trucker's chain-drive wallet. A collection of keys hung from one of the chains. Al's hair was shaved on both sides on his head, but was long in the back. On one side of his skull he sported a large tattoo, some type of bird, possibly a raven. I didn't ask. His face was decorated with multiple piercings, in his nostrils and on either side of the bridge of his nose next to each eye. I had never met anybody that looked quite like Al and I wondered how our day together was going to unfold. What was I doing here in a parking lot so far from home with somebody so different than me? What could we possibly have in common—a 26-year-old man and a 59-year-old woman? By the end of the day, that question would be answered.

Motorcycle riding is not exactly the most social of activities, despite what many riders think. It's not like traveling in a car where you can continually engage in conversation. Even if you are riding in a big group of motorcycles, you only get a chance to talk when you stop. I wondered what we would talk about when we stopped.

We exchanged greetings and Al suggested I take the lead on our ride. Our first stop was a scenic pullout overlooking Elk Lake. As the lake came into view, I couldn't help but pull off 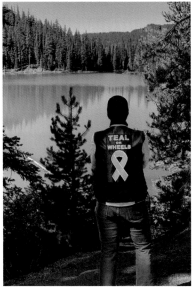 into a small parking area. The view was heavenly. We chatted for a bit and took some pictures. Al was very knowledgeable about the surrounding trees and rock formations. He pointed out some rocks that we had been riding by and told me they were actually lava from the many volcano eruptions that occurred in the Cascade Mountain range a long, long time ago. I was impressed that a young person would have such vast knowledge of nature. Al may have grown up in Massachusetts, but his heart belonged to the great

*View at Elk Lake*

outdoors. He had left home to follow his Irani girlfriend, Golnar, to the West Coast. His first job after making his cross country trip was in Bozeman, Montana working for Americorps.

We moved on from Elk Lake and passed a turn off the main roadway called Elk Loop. I thought to myself, I should have turned there, but it was too late. We continued onward. After we had traveled just a short way, I saw another turn, again it said, Elk Loop. I figured it was the opposite end of a loop road and decided that we should see where it might lead. I was hoping for another scenic vantage point of Elk Lake. I turned left off the main road and Al followed. It was a winding road that seemed to grow more narrow the further we traveled. This was not a problem for us on our bikes, but it would be if we encountered a car coming the opposite way. The road, suddenly and without warning, turned to gravel. Hard packed gravel would have been manageable, but this gravel was deep and loose with a surface some bikers would describe as riding on a washboard. My bike bounced up and down, but I was afraid if I went any slower, my bike would fall over. I looked ahead and all I could see was hundreds and hundreds of yards of more gravel roadway with no end in sight. I thought to myself, what the hell am I going to do now? I knew Al must have been thinking the same thing, especially towing that trailer behind him. Soon I was able to safely come to a stop and get my feet down. Al stopped a little ways behind me. Al, being much better with his phone than me, quickly accessed a map app and figured out where we were. He determined that we had several more miles to go on this gravel nightmare of a road. We agreed that we needed to turn around, but that was not going to be easy, especially for me on this narrow road. Making a slow speed turn in these washboard ridges of loose gravel was going to require a certain amount of luck, strength, and finesse. My Harley weighs almost 800 pounds completely loaded, so if it started to tip over in a situation like this, I probably would not be able to stop it and I would go down with the bike risking injury to me and to my bike. Al suggested he turn his rig around first. His bike would not dump because of the trailer attached and I am sure he had plenty of experience in situations like this. He struck me as an adventurous, off-road rider. He would then spot me and my motorcycle to make sure I didn't dump it and that I could safely complete the turn. That sounded like a good plan, but still my anxiety level grew. With Al's help, I successfully got the bike turned around and we hightailed it back to the paved roadway.

There are certain situations I do not care for when I am riding. They include loose gravel roads, sandy parking lots, dirt roads, mud roads, riding in hail, strong winds, lightning and pouring rain—not necessarily in that order. As a rider, you cannot control the weather and if you are an adventurous rider, you will find yourself doing a little off-roading from time to time. You have to be prepared for any situation that might arise. The more I ride, the more I learn. Experience in all riding situations matters and the only way to get that experience is to just do it and overcome your fears.

After riding a while longer, I made another stop to take some medication. When I ride, I often find myself in pain, so Ibuprofen, Aleve, Arthritis Strength Tylenol, and a roll-on Lidocaine cream all travel with me. It's the only way I can continue doing what I love. As a cancer patient, I have stronger drugs for pain, but never use them when I am riding. At this stop, a funny scenario played out in my head. Here we were, just Al and me, out in the middle of nowhere. We had barely seen any people or vehicles as we traveled along the byway. I thought to myself about how trusting I am of people. I always have been. Many of my friends expressed great concern about my safety as I was planning my Teal on Wheels ride. I had very little concern about that. I knew I would be just fine. But at this particular stop, I gave Al's trailer a longer look. I didn't know what he had inside the trailer. He said he carried camping gear, food, and other supplies. As an outdoorsman, Al spent many nights setting up camp as he traveled around the country on his motorcycle. I think he preferred to sleep under the stars rather than in a comfy hotel bed. May-

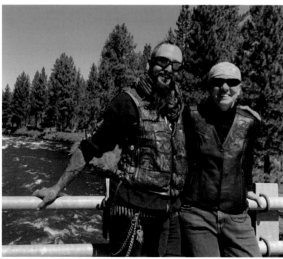

be it was a matter of economics, but I don't think so. I think he just preferred being one with nature. Anyway, I noticed attached to the outside of the trailer were several red gas cans and a shovel. I thought, Holy Crap, he could kill me, set

*Al and me at the Deschutes River*

me on fire, dig a hole, and bury me. We are out in the middle of nowhere and nobody would ever find me! That thought did not last long. There was nothing about Al to suggest he was that kind of guy. In fact, quite the opposite, everything about him suggested he was the kind of guy that might give you a kidney if you needed one.

We made several more stops throughout the day's ride enjoying the scenery and appreciating nature. At each stop, Al would ask me questions—about my cancer, about my life, and what I wanted out of life. These were serious, soul searching questions coming from a young man who I barely knew, but somehow I felt like we had been friends for years. It was refreshing to meet someone like Al and have the privilege to spend a day with him. It made me believe there was hope for Al's generation—hope for our world. Maybe there are a lot of young people like Al out there. I sure hope so. Maybe we should take the time to get to know them rather than judge them because they look different or act different than we do. Al taught me a few things that day. He taught me how to really appreciate all that is around us—to soak up nature's gifts and to be thankful for all that we have available to us. He also reinforced in me something I think I already do— talk to people you don't know. Invite someone new into your life. You might be pleasantly surprised at how taking a chance can impact your life in a positive way.

Al, thank you for spending the day with me. It was a day I will never forget.

# Chapter 8

# WHY CAN'T I BREATHE

**At my first chemotherapy appointment,** on June 16, 2016, the nurses had a hard time getting my IV started. It took four attempts. Each successive try to access my veins seemed more painful than the previous one. I was seated in one of the big, padded, reclining chairs in the Island Infusion Center. Charlie was seated next to me in a regular chair holding the hand opposite of the arm the nurse was working on. I grimaced and pursed my lips with each stab of the needle. This wasn't the way I wanted to start 18 consecutive weeks of chemo.

      Like every hospital I had ever worked in, Mount Desert Island (MDI) Hospital in Bar Harbor, where the infusion center was located, had an "expert sticker". I had worked in several hospital laboratories in my career and whenever the phlebotomist had an extremely challenging patient to stick and couldn't get the blood, a phone call back to the lab requesting the "expert" was made. Everyone working in the lab knew who that was. Even the emergency room staff and the floor nurses knew the name of the expert. She, or he, would make their way to wherever the challenging patient was located and there would be no doubt, they would be successful in their attempt to draw the blood, walking away with full tubes every time. I imagined it was the same with starting IVs. The hospital had to have an expert IV sticking nurse somewhere in the building. Sure enough, such a person existed and she was called in for the challenge. In all fairness to those who had previously tried and failed, I offered the expert my center antecubital vein, a prominent vein located at the elbow bend. There are many reasons not to put an IV in that vein and over the years of being sick, I now think I know them all. Accessing a vein lower down in the arm toward the wrist is preferable, but I know my veins well, and knew that it would be the last stick I would get that day if they used the big vein in the middle of my arm. I had been drawing my own blood for years and whenever one of my medical providers ordered any lab tests on me, I always used that center vein. It never failed me. I talked the IV sticking expert nurse into using my favorite vein for today's chemotherapy so we could finally get started.

During my chemotherapy session that day, Charlie and I discussed, and decided, that I should get a port-a-cath, or chemo port as it is commonly known. I knew I could not go through this repetitive sticking each week. A port is an implanted device consisting of a rubber septum and flexible tubing that is threaded into a vein under the skin of the chest, about an inch below the collarbone. It could stay there for years as long as it continued to work. My device was called a power port and could be used for my chemotherapy drugs, other IVs, injections during procedures like CT scans, and could even be used to draw blood. Having a port was going to make my life easier, one stick each week would yield the blood needed for lab tests before my treatment and the IV placement for fluids and my chemo drugs. After four sticks on the first week of chemo, having a port put in seemed like a no-brainer as I was beginning a regimen of four months of weekly treatments and who knew what else after that.

I was scheduled for the procedure the following week with MDI Hospital general surgeon Dr. Charles Hendricks. That was reassuring for me. Dr. Hendricks was the surgeon who performed my bowel obstruction surgery and who, by being so thorough during the surgery, had discovered the nodules on my small intestines, revealing my ovarian cancer. My port insertion was scheduled to be done in the short procedure unit on an outpatient basis, so I would be able to go home to Swan's Island once the procedure was completed. I would need to spend a little bit of time in the recovery area after the procedure, but once I was fully awake I would be able to leave the hospital. Of course, I would need a driver and that would be Charlie. The procedure for my port placement was scheduled too late in the day for us to make it home to Swan's Island on the last ferry, so we came in our own boat that we left tied to the float in Bass Harbor, next to the ferry terminal dock. We would head home whenever we got back to Bass Harbor after my procedure.

When I arrived at the short procedure unit that afternoon there were papers to sign. One was a release of liability. I remember Dr. Hendricks saying to me that there was a one percent chance of a lung puncture during the procedure. I laughed and said something like, "Dr. Hendricks, I've had such bad luck with this cancer, I can't imagine that my bad luck could continue" and assured him that I was not worried. I didn't know how wrong I was as I signed my signature on the paper.

I must have been on the verge of consciousness and unconsciousness towards the end of the procedure because I thought I had a sense of what was happening, but then I wasn't quite sure. I remember near the end of the procedure a portable x-ray machine was brought in to check the port placement while I was still in the operating room. I was then taken to the recovery area, where again, I thought I could hear voices just outside my area saying something like "she's going to be sore." I didn't know if they were talking about me or another patient. I felt like I was in some kind of fog and wasn't sure what was real.

I was eventually discharged to Charlie's care and we made our way toward Bass Harbor to go home. On the way, we stopped for a prescription of pain medication at Carroll Drug Store in Southwest Harbor. We also stopped for a pizza for the boat ride home. We got down aboard the boat and decided to eat a slice of pizza before leaving the float. It was going to be a bit of a rough crossing back to Swan's Island and we thought we better eat first and not while we were underway. I wasn't feeling very well at this point. I was in substantial pain. My chest hurt from the procedure, which had involved about a three inch incision. I decided to take one of the pain pills before we left Bass Harbor.

Our plan was to navigate to the far side of Swan's Island, about 8 miles, to Burnt Coat Harbor, instead of landing at the closest point in Mackerel Cove. We lived in Burnt Coat Harbor, but going all the way there would add about 20 minutes to our trip. As we got underway, I began to feel awful. The sea was rougher than we expected and with each wave we crossed, the boat would rise over the crest and fall hard into the troughs be-tweens the waves. I was in a lot of pain and the rough seas were not helping. Charlie decided to take me to Mackerel Cove, the closest landing point on Swan's Island, now about 20 minutes away. He would drop me off there and then take the boat around to the far side of the island to our mooring in Burnt Coat Harbor near our house. Our pickup truck was in the ferry terminal parking lot next to Mackerel Cove, so I would have to drive across the island to get home. I wasn't sure I could do it as I was now under the influence of narcotic medication, plus in a lot of pain, but I agreed to the plan.

Charlie dropped me on the float in Mackerel Cove and I slowly made my way up the ramp as he backed the boat away and changed course for the harbor on the other side of the island. I walked up the causeway from the ferry dock to the parking lot and found the pickup truck parked there. I climbed in and sat for a few minutes. Could I drive? Should I drive? I started the engine and backed out of the parking space and headed towards home.

It was a slow drive across the island, a distance of about 5 miles, but I managed to get home, park the truck in the driveway, and get into the house. Charlie would be about 30 minutes behind me getting home. He would have to put the boat on the mooring and row ashore. It was just after 7pm when I arrived home.

Over the next few hours, my pain continued to increase. I got on my iPad and Googled, "port placement and pain". I found all kinds of responses. Some patients said it was easy-peasy, nothing to worry about, very little pain involved. Other patients described varying amounts of pain, from mild to severe. I'd always thought of myself as tough—someone with a high tolerance for pain. But here I was sitting in my recliner, thinking about taking another pain pill. Was I a wimp? Had I lost my mental toughness? How would I ever get through all that was still to come in my cancer journey?

There was nothing I could do, but wait it out. I was stuck on the island for the night, with no easy way to get to the hospital in the dark. I didn't know if my condition was serious enough to warrant an expensive, after hours emergency nighttime ferry trip or if I was just being a big baby about it all. Charlie had gone to bed, but I sat up for a while longer. When I finally went upstairs and lay down my pain immediately got worse. I was having trouble breathing. Charlie was sleeping soundly and I didn't want to wake him. He had been through so much in the last couple of weeks and he needed rest. I went back downstairs and called the emergency room of the hospital where I had the procedure done just hours earlier. I thought, after hearing my story, I would be told to get the hell back to the hospital. That did not happen. I was told they would page the surgeon on call and have him call me. Unfortunately, the on-call surgeon was not Dr. Hendricks, but was someone else who knew nothing about me or the particulars of the procedure I had earlier that day. The on-call surgeon returned my phone call rather quickly and after listening to my story instructed me to come to Maine Coast Memorial Hospital in Ellsworth in the morning if I wasn't feeling any better. In just a matter of a few hours, I would soon be well acquainted with the doctor on the other end of the line. I don't remember if I got any sleep that night. I popped another pain pill and stayed sitting upright in the recliner.

When morning came, I told Charlie I felt terrible. I had had a long night of pain and discomfort sitting in the recliner. With each breath, I felt a sharp pain. I told Charlie about all the information I had learned from Google the night before and about my call to the ER and the resulting conversation with the on-call surgeon. Charlie, a trained EMT, grabbed a stethoscope from his emergency medical bag. He listened to both of my lungs. He removed the stethoscope and handed it to me and said, "You listen." He did not share his findings, but patiently waited for me to conduct a self-assessment of my lung sounds. My right lung sounded just fine. I could clearly hear the sounds of inhalation and exhalation. Then I put the stethoscope on the left side of my chest, the side that I had the surgery on the day before. I listened and listened, but heard nothing. I removed the ear pieces from my ears, turned to look at Charlie, and said, "I can't hear anything." He said, "Get your bag packed, we're going to the ER."

There was no way for me to hurry, I was operating on about half of my normal oxygen volume. By the time I got my suitcase packed, it was clear that our best bet would be to take our own boat back to the mainland. The ferry was not on Swan's Island at the time and we would have to wait for it to return from Bass Harbor. Going in our own boat would be quicker. We had left our car on the mainland the day before, so we were all set with a vehicle on the mainland to drive to the hospital. Unlike the day before, the sea was calm and we made the crossing quickly and fairly comfortably.

As Charlie was tying our boat to the float in Bass Harbor, where we had just left about 14 hours earlier, I got my suitcase and attempted to make my way up the ramp to the causeway. When I got to the top of the ramp I was gasping for air. I stopped and rested. Once the oxygen in my only functioning lung replenished, I began to walk up the hill on the ferry causeway to the ferry terminal building. I was dragging my small wheelie suitcase behind me. The terminal was not very far away, but in my condition it felt like it was a mile away, or a hundred miles. I couldn't get there. I stopped again and sat on the guardrail on the side of the causeway. Bob, the ferry terminal manager, spotted me and came rushing down the causeway. He expressed great concern and asked me what was wrong. Bob knew that I had recently been diagnosed with cancer. He lost his wife to cancer a while back and he had been especially kind to me whenever he saw me. Bob understood what I was going through. He grabbed my suitcase and helped me the rest of the way to the terminal.

## *Chapter 9*

# COLLAPSED LUNG

**As we made our way to** Maine Coast Memorial Hospital in Ellsworth, a 25-mile drive, the reality of how incredibly unpredictable this cancer journey was going to be set in. I had hopes of salvaging my summer while doing weekly chemo, but I was now feeling hopeless as my life began to spin out of control. A seemingly simple surgical procedure the day before now had me on my way to the local emergency room.

I phoned on the way there to let the ER staff know we were coming. I explained my situation and most certainly used the words, 'chest pain' in describing my current circumstances. Saying chest pain always yields an immediate response for patient care at an emergency room. We were met at the entrance where we quickly shared some basic information before I was whisked away in a wheelchair for an x-ray. I was diagnosed with a pneumothorax, more commonly known as a collapsed lung, in what seemed like a matter of minutes after arriving. A collapsed lung occurs when air leaks into the space between your lung and chest wall. It is considered a medical emergency and is usually the result of an accident, like a puncture to the lung. There are partial collapses and complete collapses. My lung was fully collapsed. The staff in the ER seemed surprised that I had been able to walk through the ER door under my own power.

I don't remember much about what happened next, only meeting the surgeon whom I'd spoken to on the phone the night before. An IV was started and I was quickly sedated. A tube, close to a half inch in diameter, was inserted into the left side of my chest wall, about four inches under my armpit. During a chest tube procedure, a hollow plastic tube is inserted between the ribs into the pleural space inside the chest. The tube is connected to a suction machine designed to help remove extraneous air from the chest and allow the lung to re-inflate. The tube stays in place until all the air is removed from the chest, typically a few days. At the site where the chest tube was inserted, my side was aggressively taped around the tube to keep any air from entering or exiting the incision site. The whole procedure was quite painful and I was given pain medication to keep me more comfortable.

My chest tube was connected to a box of bubbling water called a water seal chamber. If the box bubbles significantly it means there is an air leak. Over time, the lung should be re-expanding and the bubbling, which indicates the lung is leaking air, should become less. Once the lung has fully expanded, it is supposed to self-seal at the site of the puncture. This typically takes a few days. This was not the case for me. Day after day after day, the portable x-ray machine rolled into my room and took a picture. My lung was only partially re-inflating. Something was wrong.

I asked how long it would take for my lung to fully inflate and the doctor replied, "As long as it takes." What kind of an answer is that? I had a job, a life, and chemotherapy to get back to. I couldn't be a prisoner of this room for much longer. I was going crazy. I was tethered to that damn bubbling box by tubing that only allowed me to get out of bed and onto a bedside commode. I could not leave the room and go for a walk. I could not even get to the bathroom inside my own room. I revolted! I had a great nurse with a great name—Donna. Donna was from Steuben, Maine. She was kind, a woman with a take charge personality. She took great care of me. Donna got longer tubing and replaced the tubing on the water seal unit so that I could get to the bathroom. No more bedside commode. At least now I could have some privacy. Not only did I have the tubing from the chest tube to deal with as I moved around my room, I also had an IV in my new port for fluids and pain medication. The new port was working fine. At least something was going my way. I was also wearing a nasal cannula, tubing up my nose that provided me with oxygen. I was a tangled mess of tubing every time I rolled over in bed or tried to get out of bed.

I was in a private room with plenty of space so I asked for a treadmill or an exercise bike. I could feel that I was losing physical ability every day from just lying in the hospital bed. My health was rapidly declining. All of my requests were denied. I was considered a fall risk due to all the pain medications I was receiving. Morphine, Dilaudid, Fentynal, Oxycodone—I have no idea what I was on or how much I was taking but I accepted it each time it was offered. I was dealing with a tremendous amount of pain, not so much in my chest, but my side and my back from the way they had me taped up to prevent any leaks around the chest tube opening.

About a week into this torture, the phone in my room rang. I answered it and the voice on the other end was Dr. Hendricks. He asked me what was going on. I think he wanted to know why I was still in the hospital all this time. I told him there was talk of sending me to Bangor to a larger hospital to see a pulmonologist. I told him there was talk of lung surgery. That didn't sound right to him and he said, "I'll make some calls and find out what's going on." The next thing I knew, I was being taken downstairs, the first time I had left my room in a week. I was like a prisoner who had been in solitary confinement and now I was going somewhere, seeing something different. I was going downstairs to have some imaging done, maybe a CT scan, maybe an MRI, I don't remember, but something more than an x-ray, which I had been having done daily in my room. The imaging revealed that the chest tube was not in the proper position to do its job. I would be going to the operating room for another procedure. I woke up with a second chest tube next to the first one. The surgeon adjusted the placement of the first chest tube and inserted a second one. In the recovery room, it was determined that I now had two properly functioning chest tubes. I was now closer to getting back home, I hoped.

I was transported back to my room upstairs on a gurney and transferred back into my hospital bed. The bubbling box suction pump was hooked back up. I immediately started screaming—I was having severe chest pain. I thought I was having a heart attack. Amid the confusion, the charge nurse did a quick assessment and finally concluded that hooking up the suction was the last thing they did before the onset of my severe chest pain. She quickly disconnected it and my pain resolved. She called downstairs to talk to the doctor who had put the second chest tube in. After some discussion the cause was revealed. The pressure on the water seal chamber in my room had been set well above the normal level in an attempt to re-inflate my lung during the period that I had the first improperly positioned chest tube. Since the chest tube was not in the proper position, it didn't matter how high they turned up the suction—it was not going to work. Now that I had two properly positioned and functioning chest tubes, when they reconnected the suction to the tubes at the higher rate the pressure in my chest was so great that is caused me to scream out in pain. The pressure was turned down and reconnected to the chest tubes. This time everything seemed to be working fine. It was a horrible ordeal, but thankfully it was over fast and the pump was now functioning properly.

During all of the days I spent trapped in my room, people

came to visit me, lots of people. Some were close friends, others were neighbors from Swan's Island. Some people came to pray for me. Others came to offer support. Some brought gifts, like crossword puzzle books and adult coloring books. Some brought food. One man, a Vietnam veteran from Swan's Island, came to see me. He showed up in military boots, camo pants and his army green wife beater tank with a machete hanging on his side. I wondered how he got through hospital security with that but then I remembered I was in Maine—knives and guns are commonplace here. His name was Steve, but everyone knew him as Swanny. He brought me a bag with an apple and a piece of cake. We shared a nice conversation and our friendship grew closer that day.

My memory is not all that sharp about everyone who came to see me and what we might have talked about. After days and days of pain medication, my ability to stay sharp and focused was eroding. Depression crept in. The unknown of how long I would be hospitalized took a toll on me. But then something wonderful happened—Kyle came to see me! I was sitting in my bed one night when a man and a teenage boy came to my door. I didn't recognize the boy or the man at first and thought they were in the wrong room. Or maybe I was just hallucinating at that point and they really weren't there at all. Then the man spoke, "Donna, baby" he said in a most familiar voice. I couldn't believe it! It was my friend Kyle and his son Larkin. Kyle was part of my old volleyball group of friends from back home in Pennsylvania where I grew up and lived until 2001 when Charlie and I moved to Maine. We were part of this wonderful group of people who played competitive volleyball when we were younger. We had so many amazing times with this group of friends. I was shocked that Kyle was here standing in my hospital room doorway. I said, "What are you doing in Maine?" He replied, "We came to see you." Kyle and Larkin had driven 600 miles to visit me in the hospital. They had no other reason to be in Maine other than to see me. How is it that one person can be so lucky to have so many people who care about them? And who drives 600 miles to visit a friend in the hospital?

We had a great visit. They brought food and the game Bananagrams with them. We played several games, chatted, and

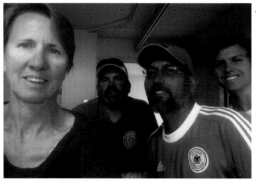 just enjoyed one another's company. Kyle's visit was a tremendous boost for my spirits. We were having a great time, but it was getting late and they had no idea where they would be staying that night, so they had to leave. They promised to come back

*Me with Charlie, Kyle, and Larkin*

the next day and see me again. Charlie was also coming the next day, so they arranged to meet at the hospital. After our second visit, Kyle and Larkin went back to Swan's Island to spend some time with Charlie.

A few days after getting the second chest tube, things started improving. My lung was re-inflating and it appeared that the puncture was sealing itself. Finally the day came for me to get out of the hospital. It was July 4th weekend. Dr. Hendricks was the surgeon on call for the two rural hospitals, so he came to see me that day and to take the two chest tubes out. I was so grateful to see a familiar and friendly face when he arrived in my room. To say the other surgeon and I did not hit it off would be an understatement, but here was my friend, Dr. Hendricks.

Getting the chest tubes out was going to be painful, but fast. Dr. Hendricks explained the procedure and instructed me on what I needed to do. He would remove them one at a time. I rolled onto my right side with the two chest tubes sticking up in the air out of my left side. My back was toward Dr. Hendricks. He removed the tape that had been holding everything together. Peeling the tape off was painful, but the worst part was still to come. He instructed me to take a breath and hold it while he pulled out the first tube. I took a breath in, held it, and he yanked on the tube. Out it came and he was right, it did hurt. I shouted out in pain. Now we had to do it one more time only this time I knew how much it would hurt. A few minutes later, the two holes in my side were bandaged and I would soon be ready to go. I asked if I could take a shower before Charlie arrived. I hadn't had a shower in 11 days and I desperately wanted one. Sponge bathing is no substitute for showering. My request was granted. Dr. Hendricks asked us to spend the night on the mainland in case I needed any further medical care. I told him we would think about it, but I just wanted to go home to the island and so we did.

My nurse Donna was the reason I kept my sanity during the long hospital stay. She worried about me like I was her own daughter. Donna was concerned about my calorie intake and would make me a Carnation Instant Breakfast milkshake with ice cream every day. One day she took all my devices away—my iPad and my cell phone, and put a sign on my door that said, "No Visitors - Please come to the nurses' station." She gave me a mirror and said, "Look at yourself. You need rest." That was probably when I felt my worst and she recognized it. One of the biggest lessons I learned from this lengthy hospital stay was something Donna told me. What she told me was that for each day you are in the hospital confined to a bed, it takes three days at home to recover. She said it would take me a month to recover from this hospital stay—a month! I didn't have that kind of time. I was resuming chemo just four days after my discharge.

*Chapter 10*

# RIDING WITH THE LADIES

**I had spent an incredible day riding** with my friend Al in the Cascade Mountains. When we parted ways, I headed east and Al went north. It was late in the afternoon when I finally rolled into Prineville, Oregon. I was hot, tired, and hungry. I saw a Best Western ahead on the left and decided it would be my resting place for the night. In my travels, I have stayed in all kinds of places, from little mom and pop motels to big chain hotels. I found the Best Westerns to be one of the best deals. I was looking forward to a comfortable and restful evening.

Per my usual routine at hotel check-in, I told the desk clerk and a trainee about my Teal on Wheels journey. I gave each of the women one of my ovarian cancer symptom cards. I could see another woman, very stylishly dressed, through an open door in an office behind the reception area. I assumed she was the manager. I gave the desk clerk another card and asked if she would give it to the woman in the office. My mission was to hand out as many ovarian cancer symptom cards as possible and I never missed an opportunity when I saw one.

I asked the desk clerk where I could find the closest entrance to my room and was told to ride down to the mid-point of the hotel and use the entrance located there. She said my room would be a short walk down the hallway from that entrance. Parking near the closest entrance to my room had become my routine each day as I unloaded my bike in the afternoon and then loaded it back up the next morning. I preferred staying at the smaller roadside motels where you could be on the first floor and park right outside your door. I was always hopeful that I would get a room where I could look out my window and see my motorcycle. That somehow made me feel better. Funny, I've never felt that way when I traveled by car.

Once the desk clerk had given me the directions to my room, I put on my helmet and rode my bike down the length of the building until I spotted the entrance. I pulled up to the curb, as close to the entrance as I could get, shut off my engine, and started my daily afternoon ritual of unloading my bike. I had only just begun the process when the very attractive woman from the office, who did turn out to be the manager, came out the door with a man in tow. My first thought was that I was in trouble for parking too close to the building and not in one of the line striped parking spaces nearby. She introduced the man as the maintenance manager and said that he had told her a woman had just checked in and was riding the same exact teal and white motorcycle that the manager, whose name was Jen, rode. When she told me that she rode and had the same bike, I had a hard time believing her. Here stood this perfectly put together woman in a form fitting dress, wearing high heels, fashionable jewelry, sassy short hairdo, and sporting perfect makeup. The last thing she looked like was a biker chick! And to think that she rode the same teal and white Harley-Davidson seemed hard to believe. However, I had met another woman earlier in the year from Massachusetts that had my same bike, so I knew it was entirely possible. We chatted for a short while about what I was doing in Prineville and about my ride across the country to raise awareness about ovarian cancer. Then we parted ways.

It was an extremely hot day and I was glad to finally get into my room and crank up the air conditioning. I was lying down on the bed trying to cool off when the hotel phone rang in my room. It startled me and seemed strange—since the popularity of cell phones, room phones hardly ever ring anymore. Besides that, who would even know I was here? I got up and answered the phone. The voice on the other end said, "Hey, it's Jen. We just met outside talking about our bikes. I was wondering if you wanted some company tomorrow on your ride?" She went on to say that her husband was out of town and that she and her friend Susie, who also rode, would be honored to ride with me the following day. The next day was the Saturday of Labor Day weekend and Jen told me she didn't have to work. I thought to myself that it might be nice to have some company for a portion of the nearly 300-mile ride I had planned for the following day. Jen seemed pleased that I agreed and said they would meet me at the hotel at 10am. I asked if they could be ready to go any earlier, but she said 10 was the earliest they could be there. We hung up and I thought to myself, what the hell am I going to do until 10am? I am usually up and gone by 7am—8 at the latest. I resigned myself to the fact that I had agreed to the departure time and that I would make the best of it in the morning by shopping for supplies at a nearby grocery store and making sure I had a full tank of gas to start the day's ride. A 10am departure even left me time to double back the way I had come into town and ride up to a scenic overlook that I passed by when I was stuck in road construction traffic. So, all in all, I would make the best of the later departure.

The next morning arrived and I had completed everything I wanted to do. I pulled my bike to the front of the hotel under the overhang and patiently waited for the ladies to arrive. I heard the familiar rumble of the Harley-Davidson engines coming down the road before I could see them. They came into view and turned into the hotel entrance. Susie was riding a white 2018 Harley Street Glide, a bike bigger and fancier than mine. Jen, who claimed the day before to have the same bike as mine, was riding a Harley Softail Deluxe. I ride a Harley-Davidson Heritage Classic, not the same bike, but similar in style. She was right about one thing though, her bike was teal and white, but it was the opposite of my bike—where I had teal, her bike had white, where I had white, her bike had teal. We got a good laugh out of it and she shared that her husband informed her the night before that she did not have the same bike as mine—not only was it not the same model, but the colors were reversed. No matter, a teal and white Harley is rare to see.

We exchanged some more pleasantries and decided to get on our way. Susie, being the most experienced rider of the three of us, volunteered to lead the ride. Jen, the least experienced, quickly offered to ride in the third position putting me in the middle of two riders I knew nothing about. I mostly ride solo, so this was not the most comfortable position for me. Riding behind Susie gave me a good vantage point to observe her riding style. She exuded confidence. She rode fast and danced in her seat to the songs playing on her bike's fancy fairing stereo system. For a while, I tried to keep up with her, but I was unfamiliar with the road and began to fall off her pace. It was a great ride filled with curves, beautiful scenery, and very little traffic. Susie's blistering pace left me feeling like I was riding out of my comfort zone. Jen stuck to me like glue—right on my tail. I decided that since she offered up her level of inexperience when we were

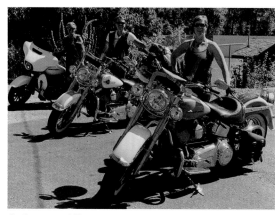

*Susie. me, and Jen*

deciding on our riding order, that the best option for the two of us was to slow down and ride at a speed we were more comfortable with. We'd eventually catch up with Susie or she'd slow down as we grew smaller in her rearview mirror. Eventually, she slowed down.

We had only been riding for about an hour when we pulled off the main highway onto a little side road that quickly landed us in the middle of downtown Mitchell, Oregon, population 124. The tiny main street was crowded with people. We backed our bikes in toward the edge of the road and got off. Susie asked what was going on. We were quickly informed that the Mitchell Labor Day parade was about to start. We strolled into a little restaurant on the main drag and bellied up to the bar. I made a hard and fast rule for myself to never drink and ride. No alcohol for me until I am off the bike for the day, so I ordered a bottle of water. My riding companions decided on beer. It was barely past 11am. I could tell at this point I was going to have to change my

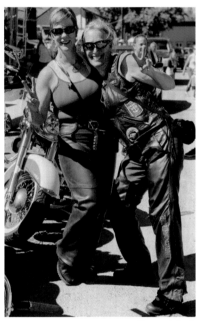

*Jen and Susie*

expectations of the distance I would be able to travel that day.

A commotion began outside. It was obvious that the parade had started. We rushed out to join in the festivities. There was no marching band and no Grand Marshall, but nevertheless it was a fun little parade with candy being thrown for the kids. Susie, who was like an overgrown child in an adult's body, dove into the street gathering up the candy and giving it to the smallest of the children standing nearby. The bigger kids were doing just fine grabbing up the candy, but the little ones needed some help and Susie obliged. Herbie the Love Bug rolled down through town, along with some various homemade floats, one titled the Mitchell Yacht Club. I imagined the nearest body of water to be hundreds of miles away and got a good laugh watching this float go by. There was even a couple of motorcycles in the parade, along with some horses and Smokey the Bear. I worried about poor Smokey. It was an extremely hot day and he must have been boiling inside that costume. I was anxious to leave as soon as the parade came to an end. There was no chance of leaving sooner as our exit route would be going against the flow of the parade and that was blocked not only by the parade itself, but also by the many spectators lining the street. We patiently waited and enjoyed the festive feel of the small town. By the time the end of the parade passed by, I was ready to get back on the bike, but we weren't going anywhere. The parade had looped around behind the little restaurant and was beginning a second lap down the main street. We were stuck watching the whole thing all over— more candy throwing, Herbie the Love Bug, the floats, and the

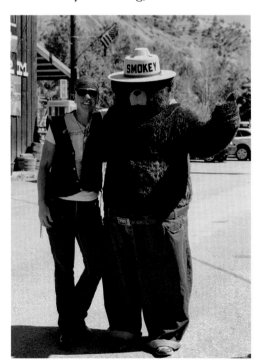

*Me with Smokey the Bear*

horses again. I ran out into the middle of the parade to get my picture taken with Smokey the Bear as he went by waving at us for a second time. At this point, I was fearful of a third or even fourth lap around the small town, but two laps concluded the parade. We were free to leave the little town of Mitchell.

We saddled up and made our way up the steep roadway dodging kids and loose dogs, running over pieces of unclaimed candy, and avoiding the horse poop left by some of the parade's equine participants. It was just a short ride back to the connection with the highway and we were soon on our way again.

We rode about another hour before Susie decided it was time to stop for some grub. I said my farewell at this point because I knew that would be at least an hour-long stop and I still had many miles to go before I could call it a day. We hugged and parted ways. It had been fun riding with Susie and Jen for the 117 miles that we covered together that day. I hope that maybe one day I will have a chance to return to the little town of Mitchell, Oregon. It was my kind of town.

## *Chapter 11*

# HEADING TO STANLEY, IDAHO

**After spending a few days** at the start of the trip exploring Oregon, it was time to push east toward Idaho. My last night in Oregon was spent in Baker City, not too far from the Idaho border. I jumped on Interstate 84 East in the morning heading toward the state line. The Snake River runs along the Oregon-Idaho border and I would soon be riding over it. My knowledge of the Snake River involved an attempt by motorcycle daredevil, Evel Knievel, to jump the river. In 1974, Knievel tried, and failed, to leap the mile-wide chasm of the Snake River Canyon on a specially designed rocket motorcycle. Forty-two years later, on September 16, 2016, stuntman Eddie Braun did what Knievel could not do. Braun successfully jumped the Canyon in a rocket motorcycle built by the son of the man who built the original rocket motorcycle for Knievel. It was named "Evel Spirit" in Knievel's honor.

Just before reaching the Snake River, I stopped at a truck stop off I-84 to fill up with gas and get some drinks and snacks for the day's ride. When I exited the convenience store, a beautiful black Harley-Davidson bagger was parked next to my bike in the parking lot. A bagger is a motorcycle outfitted with hard side saddlebags, painted to match the motorcycle's color. As I was putting my supplies in my leather saddlebags, the owner of the bike emerged from the store. He noticed my Maine license plate and asked if I had ridden all the way from Maine. I explained that I was riding across the country from the West Coast to the East Coast to raise awareness about ovarian cancer. I gave him one of my symptom cards for his wife. He asked me where I was heading that day. I told him I was heading east, across the Snake River and into Idaho. I shared that I would be heading north of Boise, up into the Sawtooth Mountains, along the Salmon River. I said, "I'm heading for Stanley, Idaho." He paused for a moment, and then told me that area was rugged country and he wasn't sure a woman, riding alone, should be heading there. He cautioned me that I would be riding long stretches where there would be no support if something went wrong. I thanked him for his concern, but despite his warning, I was heading to Stanley.

We parted ways and I jumped back onto I-84 East. I thought crossing the Snake River would feel more eventful. As I was riding across the bridge, I wondered what Evel Knievel had been thinking all those years ago. I continued on I-84 until I got to the Meridian, Idaho exit. I took Route 55 North, along the Payette River Scenic Byway. I had planned to change course after a little while and go east to Stanley, but the views along the Byway were stunning and I just kept heading north. The scenic, twisting road was a delight to ride. It was highlighted as one of the scenic motorcycle routes in my Harley Touring Handbook. It did not disappoint. The scenic valleys and distant mountains were magnificent. The road followed the Payette River and I could see people cooling off from the hot day in the river below me. There were kayaks and canoes being paddled down the river. Some bathers were floating along in big inner tubes and others were just lounging on the edge of the river enjoying the day. Before long, I arrived in Cascade, located on the scenic shore of Lake Cascade, about 70 miles north of Boise. It was late in the afternoon and I was still 144 miles from Stanley, so I decided to get a room for the night in Cascade, a small town with a population of less than 1,000. I got the last available room at the Cascade Lake Inn, a small inn located on

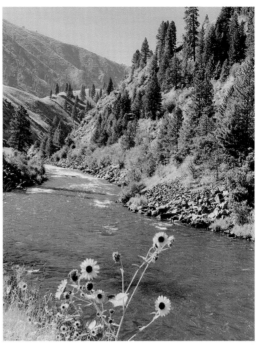

*View along the Payette River Scenic Byway*

Main Street. I pulled in the parking lot, a flat area covered with a dense bed of large, smooth stones. Immediately, I knew this surface could present a challenge for me on my bike. I chose a parking place, which wasn't really a spot at all, but a place where I knew I could pull the bike out going forward the next morning. I knew I would never be able to back my bike up on this bed of rock that made up the parking lot. One thing I always do is look for my exit before selecting a parking spot. I know better than to park my bike facing downhill—I would never be able to use my legs to push my bike backwards up a grade. I just wasn't strong enough. Any parking lots that were not paved always deserved an extra measure of caution when I entered. After safely parking, I walked into the motel office. I checked in and asked the desk clerk where I could get a burger and a beer—a place within walking distance of the Inn. She told me to head straight up the hill on the road that ran along the side of the Inn and go to the Country Club. I told her I was not interested in dining at a Country Club and she laughed, saying, "Oh, it's not that kind of Country Club at all." It was just a small restaurant called the Lakefront Bar & Grille that was located next to a golf course on the edge of Lake Cascade. I checked into my room, unloaded my bike, changed my clothes, and headed up the hill for some food.

It was a very hot day and as I was walking up the steep hill, I was feeling overheated. I couldn't wait to reach the restaurant. I stopped several times to rest, wondering how much further I had to go. I kept telling myself it would be all downhill heading back to the Inn—an easy walk home. I was hoping someone would stop and offer me a ride, but traffic was sparse and no one stopped as they drove by. Finally, I reached the crest of the hill and spotted the restaurant overlooking the beautiful Cascade Lake. The view was magnificent and well worth the trek up the hill. The restaurant was crowded and there were no tables available on the deck overlooking the lake, so I went inside and took a seat at the bar. There I met two guys, both named Joe, who were sitting at the bar. There was young Joe, sitting a few seats away. He owned a camp near Cascade and was from Twin Falls, Idaho. He came up to his camp on the weekends to go fishing. The other Joe, 76-years-old, was a local. He was seated next to me. I told both Joes that I was just passing through Cascade on my way to Stanley the next day. I shared my story about my cross country adventure. After finishing my meal and a couple of beers, I was ready to walk back down the hill. The older Joe insisted on giving me a ride. Where was he when I was trudging up that hill? I questioned the barmaid about my safety if I was to get in Joe's truck with him. She assured me that I would be safe. I said, "If there's a teal and white Harley sitting down in the parking lot at the Cascade Lake Inn tomorrow afternoon, it means Joe has killed me and left my body somewhere. Please call the sheriff." The Joes, the barmaid, and I all laughed about my statement, but secretly I thought maybe it was a possiblity. I paid my tab and out the door with "old" Joe I went. On the way out, Joe ran into some people he knew heading into the restaurant. They asked him who I was. I thought to myself, oh this is good, people that know Joe are seeing us leave together. My body might just be found.

We got in Joe's truck and instead of heading down the hill, he first took me for a little drive along the lakefront, pointing out areas of interest. We finally made our way back past the Lakefront Bar & Grille and he turned right heading down the hill towards Main Street. In a minute, we were at the stop sign next to the parking lot of the Inn. I said, "That's where I am staying. You can drop me off here." Joe wanted to show me the whole town of Cascade. I grew a little nervous, but I agreed. We turned right onto Main Street. We drove all around the town with Joe pointing out sites of interest—the town office, the community swimming center, the Cascade Medical Center and the town's library. Joe was proud of all that his town had to offer. This guy was no killer, he was just a nice man going out of his way to make me feel welcome in his little town. When we finished the tour around town, he dropped me off at the Inn. I thanked him for showing me such a warm welcome.

I had a good night's sleep in my cozy room at the Inn and when I woke up the next morning, I was excited to get on my way to Stanley. I expected it to be a short riding day, less than 150 miles to go, but knew it would be a scenic ride through expansive wilderness. On the Idaho map, in my touring guide, the road to Stanley was marked, (**may be closed in winter**). That always indicated undeveloped territory and that usually meant spectacular scenic beauty. I was looking forward to getting started. As I began loading up my bike, I realized I had a problem. My exit plan had been foiled. A pickup truck had pulled in at a 90 degree angle to the front of my bike, blocking my exit route. I would have to roll my bike backward and make a sharp turn in the loose stone. I checked out of my room and got on the bike. I was able to roll it about 12 inches backward, but that was it. I was stuck. I didn't have enough room to pull the bike forward under engine power without hitting the truck. I went inside and asked the desk clerk what room the owner of the truck was in. I would simply ask them to move the truck so I could get out. I went to the room and knocked and knocked, but no one answered. Perhaps they had walked downtown for some breakfast. I really was stuck—who knew how long before they would return. To my good fortune, a pickup truck full of young strong boys, four teenagers, or early 20-somethings, pulled into the parking lot. They piled out of the truck and went into the Inn's office. I followed them in and explained my dilemma asking them for some help. They were eager to assist. I got on the bike, one of the boys got on the front side of my bike and grabbed the forks, another got behind my bike and grabbed onto my luggage rack. Between pushing and pulling, we quickly moved the bike far enough away from the truck that I could now make a safe exit. I thanked the boys and was on my way. My time in Cascade had been memorable. I liked that little town.

As I pulled up to the stop sign to make a right hand turn onto Main Street, I realized I would be sitting there for a while. During the time I was working to get my bike free, I had noticed a steady stream of traffic coming from the north, heading south on Route 55. It was Labor Day and everyone was heading home from the three day holiday weekend. Countless pickup trucks went by towing boats, jet skis in the back, kayaks, canoes, rafts, paddleboards, you name it—anything involved in water activities filled the back of the trucks. I finally got a break in the bumper to bumper traffic and pulled out heading south. Traffic was terrible. We crawled along at a snail's pace. In a vehicle it's not such a big deal going slow, but on a motorcycle you have to maintain enough speed to keep the bike upright. If you are going too slow, the bike will fall over. To prevent that, you have to put your feet down to support the bike. I did a lot of 10 to 20 feet riding, then stopping and putting my feet down again, waiting for the traffic in front of me to start moving again. This is the absolute worst when you are riding a motorcycle. I'm always trying to find the positive in negative situations and this one had a positive—the scenic views of the Payette River running through the valley were so peaceful. It was one of the prettiest rides I had ever been on. I pulled off a number of times to stop and take pictures. I had about 35 miles to go on Route 55 South before I would turn left onto

Wildlife Canyon Scenic Byway, also known as the Banks/Lowman Road. As traffic approached the town of Banks, I could see my turn up ahead. No one was turning, they were all continuing south on Route 55. I would be happy to leave this traffic behind and get back to moving along at a moderate speed. As I started down the Wildlife Canyon Scenic Byway, I could see smoke up ahead. Just three days earlier, on August 30, this area between Banks and Lowman, had been the site of a wildfire. There were still fire crews on scene dousing some areas.

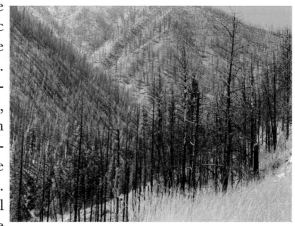
*Devastation from the wildfires*

Earlier, in July 2019, a large part of the area I was riding through had been devastated by wildfires. I was unsure if it would be safe to ride across the remote land. Maybe that guy back at the truck stop in Oregon was right—this was rugged country.

I continued on, knowing I was only about 100 miles from Stanley. If the fire danger became too great, I would turn around and find another route. For some reason, Stanley, Idaho had been on my list of places to see, despite knowing nothing about it. I just had to get there. I saw lots of burned areas on my way, but no more smoldering areas. It was sad to see the devastation left behind by the wildfires.

When I reached the town of Lowman, I turned left to go north on Route 21. This would take me the rest of the way to Stanley. I was now traveling along the edge of the Sawtooth National Recreation Area and the scenery was incredible. The Sawtooth Mountain Range is part of the Rocky Mountains. It is located in central Idaho and reaches a maximum elevation of 10,751 at the summit of Thompson Peak. The last 70 miles of my ride were indeed through some rugged terrain. I passed only one car and one motorcycle in that 70 mile stretch. I saw more elk crossing signs than anything else. I thought about an elk-motorcycle collision. That didn't sound like it would turn out too good for me, so I kept my eyes scanning the sides of the road. Back home in Maine, I often worried about deer jumping out in front of my motorcycle, but here it was elk. I never did see an elk on this stretch of roadway, although I think I would have liked it if I did. I had encountered elk just about a week earlier on my first day of riding in The Redwood National Forest, but saw none in Idaho.

It seemed like I had been riding for a long while before I began my decline out of the mountains. I spotted the town of Stanley in a valley down below. I was glad to be coming to the end of my riding for the day. I had encountered a couple of surprisingly strong wind gusts that came out of nowhere up in the mountains. One caught me off guard and threw me out of my lane and into the oncoming lane of traffic. No worries—no one was coming, but it was an uncomfortable feeling. There was a car behind me, probably someone heading for Stanley, like me. Even though I could see Stanley ahead in the distance, it was still miles away. As I made my final approach, I rolled down into the town and was greeted by a sign that read: Stanley, Idaho - Population 63. Population 63—holy crap! I had no idea the town would be so sparsely populated. I wondered if I would even be able to find a room for the night.

Despite Stanley's remoteness, it was a town built around tourism. I found several lodging options and chose the largest of the places in town to stay, the Mountain Village Resort. The Resort had its own restaurant and just across the road, a gas station and small grocery store—a whole complex of everything I would need. I unpacked my bike, taking off both of my travel bags, dumped everything in my room, and went out for a ride to explore the little town. It felt funny riding my motorcycle without all of the extra gear on it. My first stop was the Salmon River that ran right through Stanley. The Salmon River offered up some exciting fishing opportunities. Outside of town, the Middle Fork and Upper Main Salmon Rivers offer a wide variety of fish species. Stanley is the home base of many fishing outfitters. As I walked along the river, I met a family, who

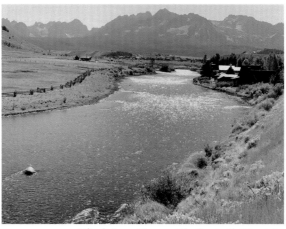

*The Salmon River and the Sawtooth Mountains*

were just introducing their young children to fishing.

Stanley is also a great jumping off point for hiking. Some of the best backpacking and climbing exist around the area. Hundreds of high mountain lakes are connected by marked trails that start just minutes from town.

I rode back the way I had come into town to take some pictures of the Sawtooth Mountains in the distance. The elevation of Stanley is 6,253 feet. I wondered how high up I was in the mountains earlier that day. I was becoming obsessed with elevation. Back home in Maine, I live at sea level, so riding in the mountains was fascinating for me. I loved keeping track of the elevation of places I was riding.

I headed back to the Resort and decided to walk next door to the adjacent restaurant and saloon. I went in the door that led to the saloon and got a seat at the bar. I began talking to a couple sitting near me. They asked me if I had been riding a teal and white motorcycle earlier that day. I was surprised that they asked. I said, "Yes, I was." The husband asked me about the big gust of wind that threw me to the other side of the road up in the mountains. They had been in the car that was following me when that happened. The man said, "That gust practically blew our car off the road." I laughed and commented on how that wind had just come up out of nowhere and that my riding had been very comfortable until that happened.

Everywhere that I traveled I met the nicest people. My trip was off to a great start and I couldn't imagine how it would get any better, but it would. The remoteness of the West was beyond anything that I had imagined. The grandness of the mountain ranges and the raw beauty of the scenery was beyond my wildest dreams. This was going to be a trip of a lifetime.

When I awoke the next morning, it was 37 degrees, too cold to saddle up and head out of town. I decided to go soak in a hot spring. The Resort had a small building down a footpath, about 150 yards away that had a hot spring running into it. The building sat right on the edge of the river and had a hot tub that was fed by the hot spring. I called the front office and asked if I could go for a soak. When I checked in the day before, the clerk told me about the hourly soaks, starting at 7am, that were available at no charge to guests. I wasn't interested at the time—it was over 90 degrees when I had arrived and the last thing I wanted to do was soak in a hot tub. But, now it was 37 degrees and it seemed like a great way to spend some time. The desk clerk told me I had to come over to the office to get a towel and sign a liability release. He said I could go down at 8am, since the 7am soak had already started and you could only go on the hour. Only eight people could go at the same time. A few minutes before 8am, I bundled up, my swimming suit was my bottom layer, Under Armour cold running leggings for my legs, a sweater, a hat, gloves and a jacket and my Keen sandals on my feet. I headed to the office, signed the release, and got my towel. I headed down the trail to the small outbuilding on the river's edge. It was very chilly on my walk down, but I passed people coming up the trail, wearing nothing but a bathing suit and towel. I said, "Aren't you cold?" They had been soaking in the hot tub and reported they were nice and warm. I was the first to arrive at the building for the 8am soak. Inside was a big concrete tub with sand in the bottom. Benches lined the inside of the octagonal tub. Steam was coming off the water. A double barn door was opened on one end of the building, near the tub, overlooking the river and

the Sawtooth Moun-
tains in the distance.
The sun was brightly
shining and the view
out the doors from
the inside of the tub
was simply stunning.
I slowly climbed
down into the pool
of water—it was very
hot, but my body
quickly adjusted to
the temperature. It
was delightful. No
other guests made an
appearance for the
8am soak time, so I

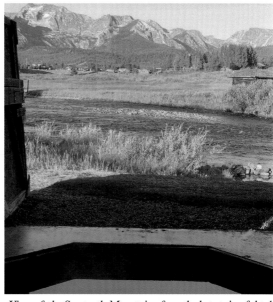

*View of the Sawtooth Mountains from the hot spring fed tub*

had the whole place to myself. It was simply heavenly, one of the
best experiences of the trip. The 7am soakers were right—when
I walked back to my room in my wet bathing suit and towel, I was
not cold at all. This was a great start to my day.

The air temperature was slowly rising. I showered, got
dressed for a cold ride, and loaded up my bike. I would be riding
south on Route 75, the Sawtooth Scenic Byway toward Ketchum
and Sun Valley Ski Resort, an area known for terrific winter ski-
ing in Idaho. Before I would reach Ketchum, I would need to
ride over the Galena Summit, a high mountain pass at an elevation of 8,701 feet. The pass, located in the Boulder Mountains,
was within the Sawtooth National Recreation Area. Located on
Route 75, about 40 miles south of Stanley, it is one of the highest paved mountain roads in Idaho and among the most iconic
climbs in the state. A little more than one mile west of the summit is Galena Overlook, a scenic viewpoint at 8,400 feet

Under the category of "Isn't it a small world," I met a
couple at the Galena Overlook and shared my story of riding my
motorcycle across the country to raise awareness about ovarian

cancer. I told them I was riding home to Swan's Island, Maine, thousands of miles away. The woman told me that many years ago her sister had been a teacher on a small island in Maine—an island

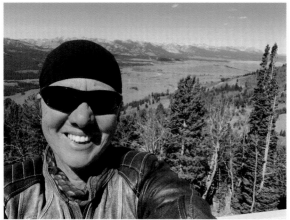

called Frenchboro. Imagine their surprise when I told them I lived three miles by water from Frenchboro and visited there several times every summer.

I continued down Galena Pass traveling south toward Ketchum

*View at the Galena Overlook*

and on toward Twin Falls. It turned into a hot ride that day. I started the day at 37 degrees when I woke up in Stanley and finished the day of riding at 92 degrees in Burley, Idaho, just north of the Utah border.

My destination for the next day's ride was Salt Lake City, Utah. I had a couple days of highway riding ahead. I would be taking I-84 South into Utah. Charlie would be flying into Salt Lake City to join me for three days of riding in southern Utah. We would have a long day of highway riding from Salt Lake City to Zion National Park the day after he arrived. I was looking forward to seeing Charlie and looking forward to visiting Zion National Park, but I was not looking forward to two consecutive days of highway riding. The reward would come when we reached Zion in two days.

## Chapter 12

# BEING BALD

**It's funny how a man can shave his head** and women think, wow, there's a sexy man, but if you see a bald woman you think, she must have cancer, poor thing. For women, hair is a big part of their identity. Women spend hundreds of dollars a year going to fancy salons for haircuts and coloring. Lots of money is spent on shampoos and conditioners, detanglers, mousse, styling gels, hair shining products, hairspray, and more. Over the course of a year, how much time is spent by women doing their hair? Blow drying, flat irons to straighten curly hair, curling irons to give straight hair more body. Whether we are getting ready to go to work, out for a date, or preparing to be on a Zoom conference—so much time is spent trying to get our hair to look perfect, or maybe for some of us, just trying to get it to look good enough. Endless hours in front of the mirror and endless amounts of money spent trying to achieve the perfect look. Why all this fuss over our hair, ladies?

I envy men and their hair styles. My husband Charlie spends 99 cents on a bottle of VO5 shampoo. He might own a can of mousse, but I'm not sure he ever uses the stuff.

For many women, hair is important—it's part of who we are. So the fear of losing all of your hair during chemotherapy is terrifying. Your body is already under an attack by your cancer, and an additional assault by your chemo drugs—then you lose all your hair. For those of you who don't know, it is not just the hair on top of your head—it's all your hair. There are some advantages to that, you don't have to shave your legs or your armpits. No more plucking your eyebrows or those stray chin hairs. But the advantages do not even come close to making up for the bigger angst of walking around bald—for almost a year!

Being bald does give you the opportunity to try a new hairstyle if you get a wig. You could try a few fun wigs in different styles and colors. If a wig is not your thing, you could buy some pretty scarves and learn how to tie them so they look just right. Or you can fall back on the easiest remedy, wear a baseball cap to cover up your baldness. It's a personal choice, but none of those solutions were right for me.

When my hair started to fall out, exactly 14 days after my first chemo treatment, just like I had read, I was stuck in the hospital with a collapsed lung and couldn't do a thing about it. I had leaned over the bathroom sink to wash my hair and globs and globs of strands of hair covered the drain by the time I was finished. Even though I had been warned, it still came as a shock to me. It was awful, my scalp was painful. I had a trash can next to my hospital bed and I found myself gently tugging on handfuls of hair and out it would come. I couldn't stop myself. At this point, I just wanted it all gone.

When I finally got discharged from the hospital, Charlie took me to see my hairdresser, Kim. I had been to see Kim a few weeks earlier when I had her cut my hair fairly short before I was set to start my chemo treatments. I thought that might make the transition to baldness easier when it all fell out. This time I said to Kim, "Shave it off." I still had quite a bit of hair left—strands of short thinning hair. If the wind blew my hair just right, bald spots were revealed. Kim asked, "Three-quarter inch, half inch, or quarter inch?" I picked the half inch. Kim got her clippers and it didn't take her long before all my remaining hair, except for a half inch of fuzz, was laying on the floor. It was a relief really. There wasn't a thing I could do with the straggly array of thinning hair that remained on the top of my head,

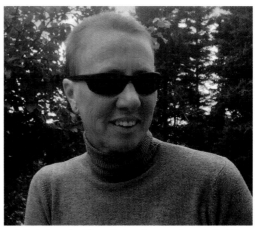

*My haircut by Kim - before the rest of my hair fell out*

so now it was gone. I asked Kim how much I owed her and she said, "Nothing." She hadn't charged me for the haircut a few weeks earlier either. I tried to argue with her that she couldn't stay in business giving away haircuts. She said, "It's the least I can do for you, Donna." Kim was among the many angels who revealed themselves during my cancer journey.

We left the salon and headed home. On the ferry ride to Swan's Island, I found myself just rubbing my head, checking out my new haircut. It felt fuzzy, yet soft. I liked the feel. When I got home I stared at my new haircut in the mirror. I'd worn my hair short for most of my life, but never this short. I thought to myself, I kind of like this. There had never been anything special about my hair. It was straight and thin and for years I had it colored. I didn't even know what my real color was anymore. I had often thought about not coloring it, but I couldn't figure out how I would let it grow out without having two distinct colors until I could get all the colored part cut off. My problem was now solved. When it grew back I would just keep my natural color—whatever that was. I had no idea how long it would take for my hair to grow back once I was finished with my chemotherapy, maybe a few months, maybe closer to a year.

I had decided that I wasn't going to get a wig and I couldn't picture myself with any fancy scarves. I didn't much care for wearing ball caps. I landed on skull caps, lightweight hats that covered your skull, like the little hats some NFL football players wore under their helmets. My neighbor Leah crocheted a couple of hats for me in pretty blue colors. I wore them when it was cooler, in the early morning. Some days I would make a hat out of a BUFF by twisting it in half and folding it back on itself. This gave me some hats with fun colors and prints. I was having my treatment through the summer months and wearing a hat was hot. After a while I decided the easiest thing to do was just go around bald. After all, who was I trying to fool? Everyone knew I was bald and I imagined they were curious about it. So I put away all the head coverings and went about my business with my head in an au natural state—completely bald. The half inch of hair that my hairdresser had left eventually fell out, too, leaving me as bald as a cue ball.

I remember being at an appointment in Bar Harbor with Charlie where we would be seeing Dr. Philip Brooks, one of my oncologists. We were patiently sitting in the waiting room with a few other patients. I was there in all my bald gloriousness—the only bald woman in the waiting room. I leaned over to Charlie and whispered, "Should I put on my hat?" He nodded yes. I sensed he might be uncomfortable with my looks, but because he nodded yes, I chose not to put my hat on. I can be a bit defiant at times.

I started my chemo on June 16, 2016 and my hair started falling out on June 30. I had my hair shaved off a week later, on July 7, when I got out of the hospital. I stopped my chemo on September 2. I wondered how long it would take for my hair to grow back. I checked with other ovarian cancer patients on Inspire.com, an online cancer community I had joined. It seemed like everyone had a different experience. It was not as cut and dry as the 14-day time period for your hair to fall out. I was anxious for my hair to grow back, but I would just have to wait. It would happen when it happened.

The morning sun shone brightly through a big picture window that my kitchen table sits up against. Charlie sat on one side of the table and I sat directly opposite from him. For weeks, each morning I would lean across the table and ask him if he could see any growth. Every morning he would say no and I would lean back and sit back down in my chair, disappointed. I was worried that my hair would never grow back. One morning after he said no again for what seemed like the hundredth time, he said, "Wait a minute. Lean over here again." So I did. This time he said he could see something. I asked Charlie what color it was and he replied, "White." Oh no, my real hair color was going to be white? Had I turned grey and didn't know it?

As my hair slowly started to grow, there was some grey in it, but mostly it was dark. But the most surprising thing was that it was curly. I'd always had poker straight, fine hair. As my hair grew and grew, it got curlier and curlier. I liked this new style, but it was not going to last. When I finally got my first haircut, just to neaten up the mess on my head, the curls were gone. I learned that the chemo drugs not only attack the cancer, but every other

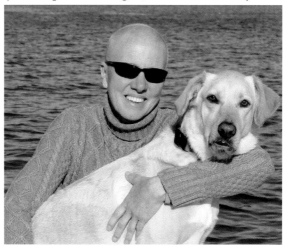

*Hanging out with Roscoe - 6 weeks after stopping chemo*

cell in your body, including cells in the hair follicles. It takes a while after finishing chemo for the drugs to leave your system. The change in the hair follicles are what causes hair to grow back differently. Changes in texture and color can occur. For me, it didn't matter what my hair looked like, just as long as it was coming back.

The trauma of losing all my hair was not as great as it is for many women. I've never had beautiful hair, so it was not, and is not, a big part of my identity. After my initial shock, I actually found that the time that I was bald to be easier for me. Fixing my hair was one less thing I had to deal with during a very challenging time in my life.

# Chapter 13

# UTAH...LIFE ELEVATED

**I had only set foot in Utah once before,** spending less than 5 minutes in the state. Back then, I was there just long enough for Charlie and me to jump out of our friend Mike's car, run up to the "Welcome to Utah" sign, and get our picture taken. We hopped back in the car, Mike turned around, and we drove back across the state line and into Arizona. When I arrived in Utah this time, it was a very different experience. I would spend 5 days there and it still was not enough time to take in all that this amazingly beautiful state had to offer.

During the planning of the trip, I had imagined my time in Utah to be some of my best days riding. Southern Utah was my ultimate destination. There, I would visit Zion, Bryce Canyon, and Arches National Parks. Riding through the parks and surrounding areas would be amazing, or at least that's what I was envisioning.

Charlie had been so supportive of me making this trip and I felt like I wanted to be able to not only share my photos and stories with him, but I wanted to share some of the riding with him, too. I asked him to meet me in Salt Lake City when I got there and go with me on part of my trip. He arranged his flights to and from Maine and reserved a rental motorcycle for pick up in Salt Lake City. We would ride southern Utah together.

I needed to arrive in Salt Lake City eight days after the start of the trip to meet Charlie when he arrived. I had already ridden 1,554 miles by the time I got there. When I was up in Stan-

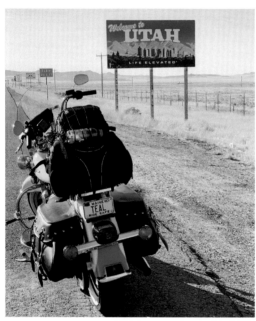

ley, Idaho, I had hoped to go further north to Yellowstone National Park in Wyoming, but I didn't have enough time to get there and back to Salt Lake City in time. Scratching Yellowstone off my list was hard, but it was going to be necessary if I was going to be able to rendezvous with Charlie as planned. He would be flying into Salt Lake City from Portland,

*Welcome to Utah...Life Elevated*

Maine. A rental motorcycle would be waiting for him at the Eagle Rider location near the airport. We would spend the night in Salt Lake City and get an early start the next morning riding south, about 300 miles, to Zion National Park. It all sounded good when we made our plans, but a storm, with hurricane force winds on the East Coast, forced the cancellation of his flight from Portland. He took a bus to Boston where he would be able get a flight out the following day. The delay in his departure meant he wasn't going to be able to meet me on the afternoon of September 4 as planned. If all went well, he would arrive around noon the following day. After much back and forth discussion we decided that I would leave for Zion as planned and ride the 300 plus miles alone. It was hot in Utah and I wanted to try and beat the heat of the middle part of the day by leaving early. Hopefully, Charlie's flight would arrive by noon, he would pick up his rental bike, and be about 5 hours behind me, arriving at our planned destination no later than 6pm.

His late arrival in Salt Lake City was not a complete bust. A dear friend, Bryan, was traveling across the country from Arizona to Washington, DC and happened to have a multi hour layover in Salt Lake City. We arranged to meet at my hotel and go out for dinner. After his plane landed, Bryan got an Uber to the hotel. It was nice to see a friendly face standing at the door of my hotel room and he was wearing a Teal on Wheels T-shirt. My friend Denise had gotten the shirts made as a fundraiser for my trip and I had no idea who had ordered one. Obviously, Bryan's wife, Janelle, had ordered them for the whole family. Bryan and I walked to a nearby pub for dinner. If I couldn't enjoy dinner with Charlie that night, Bryan was the next best thing.

I left Salt Lake City the next morning in the middle of rush hour and hopped onto Interstate 15 South. The traffic was horrendous. Six lanes of white knuckle riding, with road construction through most of the busy Salt Lake City traffic. Lanes were shifting left and right to accommodate the ongoing construction, but the newly painted temporary lines were difficult to see. I was stuck in the inside lane and could see an express lane on the far outside that allowed single occupancy drivers and motorcycles to travel at a much faster speed. There was a fee you had to pay to travel in that lane and that was not a problem at all. The problem was that I could see no way to safely move across five lanes of speeding trucks and cars. I could not find a gap in the heavy traffic that would allow me to exit my lane and into the next and the next and the next, so I stayed riding in the inside lane with on ramps and exits presenting even more challenges. It was the most stressful riding of the trip so far. I was pretty sure that once I got south of Provo, the highway traffic would be less and it would also be past rush hour by then. I hunkered down, gritted my teeth, and hung on tightly to my handlebars. I was on hyper focus mode watching for any erratic drivers, ready to react quickly to the circumstances around me. Not only was the traffic awful and the roadway poorly marked, but the speed at which these rush hour commuters were driving made my head spin. In the urban areas, the speed limit was 70 mph. In the rural areas, the maximum speed limit on I-15 was 80 mph, a bit faster than I normally cared to ride, but I thought it would help me make good time covering the 300 miles I had to ride that day.

My destination for the night was an Under Canvas Glampground, one of the luxury campgrounds that are popping up across the country. A few months earlier, on Swan's Island, Jamie, a representative from Under Canvas, had come to the island to talk with my community members about the company she worked for building a high-end camping operation on a piece of shoreline property. Swan's Island's close proximity to Acadia National Park was the draw for Under Canvas. It seemed like all of their luxury campsites were located near National Parks. I liked the idea of a glampground on Swan's Island and thought it would be an economic boost for my community. I was supportive of hearing more about the proposal, but the majority of the voting members of my community were not in favor. After receiving very little support at the meeting, I invited Jamie back to our house for a few beers. She accepted my offer. When we first arrived at my house, I took Jamie to my garage to see my motorcycle and told her about my upcoming cross country trip. She shared information with us about the whole glamping culture and mentioned that Under Canvas had several glamping locations in southern Utah, near the National Parks we planned to visit. After Jamie's departure, we continued to communicate and she offered several nights of complimentary accommodations in Utah. I gladly accepted her offer and settled on two nights, one at the Under Canvas Zion location and another night at Under

Canvas Moab, adjacent to Arches National Park. I was excited to experience outdoor luxury camping and was looking forward to my arrival that afternoon.

It was a blistering hot day of riding. Temperatures rose from the 80s at the start of the trip, into the 90s by early afternoon, and topped 100 degrees by the end of the ride. I stopped several times along the way to take a break and hydrate. Some motorcyclists use the acronym ATGATT, which stands for all the gear, all the time. It means you commit to wearing all the safety gear every time you ride. I was a firm believer in this, but found that when the riding temperatures climbed out of the 80s and into the 90s, it was no longer possible to keep all your gear on. The safety gear consisted of a leather jacket, helmet, gloves, and leather chaps—it was enough to cause you to have a heat stroke. I was sweating profusely and couldn't take in enough fluids on my short stops. I had to lose my leather jacket and was down to riding in just a T-shirt and jeans. I hadn't put my leather chaps on that morning—I knew it was going to be too hot for them. I always wear a helmet, no matter what, but now wished I had a white helmet instead of a black one, or a vented helmet that would at least let in some air. I made several stops along the way. The last one was a little gas station convenience store in Virgin, UT, just miles from my final destination. I stocked up on cold drinks and snacks. I was looking forward to reaching the glampground, getting off the bike, getting out of my jeans, and enjoying a cold drink. I departed Virgin and took the Kolob Terrace Road, a mountainous road with exquisite views that led me to Under Canvas Zion, situated just on the western edge of Zion National Park. There was no development, no houses, only spacious open land surrounding the glampground offering spectacular views in every direction.

I pulled off the paved roadway and into the entrance of Under Canvas. It was a hard-packed dirt road with loose gravel on top in some spots. It was windy and hilly and I did not like the look of it or the feel of it under my tires. I guess I had not thought to ask if it was appropriate to arrive on a motorcycle. My off-road riding skills were about to be tested. I made my way up and down the rugged road following the reception area signs with arrows guiding me to a large main tent that housed the reception desk and restaurant. I parked my bike and entered the tent. I was completely overheated when I arrived and very quickly an employee inside the reception area opened the lid on a large cooler filled with cold, wet wash clothes and offered me one. I gladly accepted and wiped the sweat off my face first and then placed the cool cloth on my neck. It provided a refreshing relief from the heat of the day. I checked in and found out that Jamie had made arrangements for us to stay in a deluxe tent with a king sized bed, ensuite bathroom, private deck, and a wood burning stove. Ha, we would not be needing the stove, but air-conditioning would have been welcome. The temperature when I arrived was 106 degrees.

I followed a staff member, driving an electric powered golf cart, to my tent. A small parking place in front and off to the side offered enough space for one car, or conveniently, two mo-

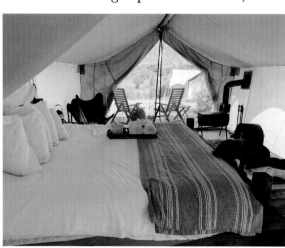

torcycles. I pulled into the spot, being sure to leave enough room for Charlie to park when he arrived in a few hours. The staff person removed a large cooler filled with ice from the back of the golf cart and placed it on the deck leading into

*Inside our deluxe tent*

the tent. She accompanied me into the tent to show me around. The tent was lovely and spacious inside. There was a king-sized bed and a few chairs for sitting. It had a bathroom inside the tent that was separated from the bedroom by a large curtain. The bathroom had a toilet, sink, and a shower. Under Canvas strives to minimize its impact on the environment and is an extremely green operation, so I was instructed on how to use the pull-chain shower to minimize water usage. There was no electricity in the tent, so I was provided with rechargeable batteries with USB ports that we could use to charge our phones and computers. On either side of the bed, there were battery operated lamps and fans. I was instructed on how the misting system worked. I turned on the misters on the outside deck, sat directly under them, and began to feel cooler—it almost felt like air conditioning. I

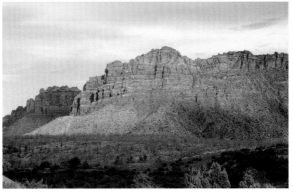

*View from the deck of our tent*

had changed out of my riding gear, gotten a quick shower, and put on a skirt, tank top, and flip flops. The view from the deck of our tent was unbelievable. I imagined vacationers from urban areas arriving and thinking, WOW, just WOW! I live in a rural area, which offers an equally beautiful view of the ocean—very different from this view.

As I began to cool off, I wondered how much longer it would be before Charlie arrived. I sat in one of the chairs on the outside deck enjoying the view, relaxing, rehydrating, and reliving the trip so far.

I could see the road I had arrived on off in the distance. I don't think a single car went by as I sat on the deck. I knew I would be able to see Charlie coming from a long way off. I kept glancing in the direction he would approach from hoping to spot him. Finally, I saw a small object coming. I could see it was a motorcycle, so it had to be Charlie. I was so relieved. He had endured two long days of interrupted travel to get from Maine to Utah: car, bus, airport shuttle, plane, cab, and finally motorcycle. I'm not sure if I would have gone through all of that for three days of riding. I think I would have turned around and gone back home to the island after learning my flight from Maine was cancelled, but he forged on and now he was in the last mile of his long trek. He turned into the entrance of Under Canvas Zion and made his way to our tent site. It was great to finally be reunited. We compared stories about our rides from Salt Lake City to southern Utah. I had ridden 305.8 miles to get there. Charlie, a little less, based on his starting point. We both complained about the oppres-

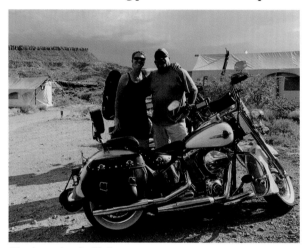

*Together at last in Utah*

sive heat. Charlie shared that he had ridden through some rain on his ride. I was envious and would have welcomed some rain on my ride that day. We couldn't believe that the speed limit was 80 mph once we got south of Pro-

vo. The road surface was great and you could see for miles on either side of the highway, giving me the confidence to ride faster than I normally do. It provided Charlie the means to make the 300 mile trip, despite an early afternoon departure, and still arrive in time for dinner.

Charlie unpacked his bike and he rested for a while before we walked up to the small restaurant at the reception tent. We enjoyed a nice meal on an outdoor patio overlooking the magnificent sandstone cliffs surrounding Under Canvas. Tomorrow, we would ride our motorcycles through Zion National Park. We could hardly wait.

*Chapter 14*

# THE THREE BIG PARKS

**As we packed up our bikes** and pulled away from our tent site at Under Canvas Zion, the sun was shining brightly. It was going to be another hot day of riding. We headed down the road toward Springdale, UT and the entrance to Zion National Park. Just a short way into the trip, we came upon a big cow grazing on some grass along the side of the road. She had slipped out of a nearby fenced in field and looked just as happy as could be. I was startled to see such a big animal standing along the side of the road. This was just the first of many encounters with cattle in Utah. Every county in the state has areas of open range, meaning the cattle can roam at will. This was something we did not know when we arrived in southern Utah, but we soon became aware of it. Back home in Maine, it was deer, and sometimes moose, that you had to look out for. I've had my share of deer jumping out in front of me at home—both in my car and on my motorcycle, but I had never encountered a cow in Maine.

This day and the next few days were going to be special—riding with Charlie and sharing part of my trip with him was something I had been looking forward to. Added to that, on this day, September 6, 2019, we were celebrating our 28th wedding anniversary. How we had managed to make it this far together was a testament to who we both were and how we dealt with adversity. We were both fiercely independent, but when we worked together toward a common goal, we could get things done. Our marriage was built on mutual respect and love. And most of all—trust. That trust allowed us to each be our own person and pursue individual dreams as well as shared goals. Charlie was not a motorcycle rider when I got my first motorcycle. He really wasn't all that interested in riding. Then I bought my second bike, and a third. It was at that point that he got his motorcycle license, but still he did not buy a motorcycle. But what he did do was encourage me to pursue my passion. I never would have taken my first big solo ride to Canada to ride the Cabot Trail if it wasn't for Charlie. The morning I was supposed to leave there was rain in the forecast. I did not get on the first ferry leaving Swan's Island, then the second ferry left. At this point, Charlie said, "Get on your bike and go or you will never leave." He was right. I left on the next ferry and nineteen miles into my 1,800 mile trip it started to rain. There was no turning back now. I had started the trip and I was going to finish it. I really had no business going on a trip like that alone. I just didn't have enough riding experience at the time. But by the time I returned home I had ridden through pouring rain, unbelievable winds, miles and miles of grooved cut pavement on roads that were under construction, and cold temperatures. I survived it all. I gained a tremendous amount of confidence and found that being on the road alone was empowering—it was something that I really enjoyed. I have Charlie to thank for his unending support for my love of riding.

Back to Utah. After a short ride, we arrived in Springdale and made our way to the toll booth at the entrance to Zion National Park. We rolled up behind some other bikers and waited our turn to enter. I already had a Lifetime Pass to all National Parks in my possession, but Charlie would need to purchase a Park Pass. He bought an annual pass that would gain him entrance not only to Zion, but also Bryce Canyon and Arches National Parks the following two days. He would also be able to use that pass the following summer back home at Acadia National Park in Maine.

In 2019, Zion National Park had over four million visitors. Traffic moved slowly as we entered the park on Route 9, also known as the Mount Carmel Scenic Highway, a 12-mile roadway connecting the South entrance with the East entrance of the park. Just after we entered, we were met with tall red canyon walls that towered over us as we rode along the switchbacks up the steep mountain road. It was hard to keep your eyes on the road with all the amazing scenery surrounding us. It was simply stunning. Near the top of Mt. Carmel was the Zion-Mt. Carmel tunnel, a 1.1 mile narrow roadway through the mountain. We traveled

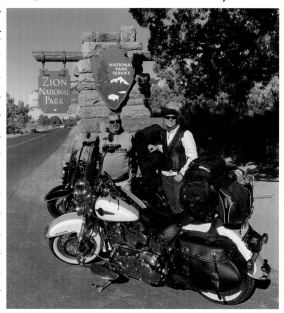

*At the East entrance to Zion National Park*

through it three times that day. If large campers or trucks were coming through the tunnel, traffic traveling the opposite direction was stopped. This caused a bit of traffic congestion, but it wasn't long before we got going again and I certainly would not have wanted to meet a large vehicle coming the other way inside the narrow tunnel. It was extremely dark inside the tunnel and I

129

had difficulty seeing. The headlights on my Harley were not very bright. There were several areas along the tunnel where the rock was carved away creating openings like windows that let the sun filter in. That helped a lot and I was glad when we got to those spots. I was wearing my prescription sunglasses, which made it even darker, but without them, I couldn't see much at all, so it was either darker from the glasses or blind without them. The ride through the tunnel was challenging. Charlie was in the lead and I just focused on the red taillight on his bike to guide me through. His rental bike was brand new and the headlights were much brighter, so he had the lead.

We rode across to the East entrance, stopping at pull-offs along the way to take pictures. The views were magnificent.

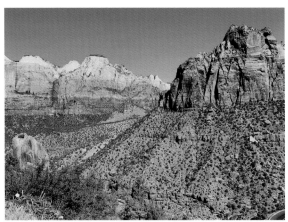

*One of the many scenice views inside Zion N.P.*

We saw some big-horn sheep high up on the cliffs. We turned around at the East entrance and rode back to the South entrance. We parked the bikes in a lot there and took a ride on a shuttle bus. The shuttle bus was the only way to visit another part of the park called Zion Canyon during the busy tourist season. Private vehicles were not allowed to go to that part of the park. We sat in the back of the bus as it traveled along the Zion Canyon Scenic Drive. We looked out the windows as the driver narrated the various landmarks along the way. There were many stops, where passengers could get off to go on various hikes, or to the Zion Lodge for lunch. Some passengers embarked as others who were waiting got on the bus. Charlie and I chatted about how much better seeing this part of the park would be from the seat of our motorcycles and not from inside on this hot bus.

By the time we returned from the shuttle bus ride, we were ready to get on our bikes and head out of the park for an anniversary lunch. Our friend Mike, from Phoenix, AZ, had recommended a small Mexican Restaurant named Oscar's Cafe located in the middle of the charming town of Springdale. We made our way to Oscar's, which had an outdoor dining patio, but we opted for a table inside so we could soak up some of the air-conditioning. We had an enjoyable lunch and mapped out our way to Kanab, where we would be spending the night. At lunch, we realized we had to go back into the park and through the dark tunnel again to get to Route 89 on the East side of the park. We'd be riding back across Route 9 again, getting a second chance to ride the switchback up Mount Carmel and enjoy the fantastic views one more time before leaving this beautiful National Park.

We made our way across the park and south to Kanab, just four miles north of the Arizona border. We had only ridden 90 miles the day we visited Zion, but it was 90 spectacular miles. The next day we would be visiting Bryce Canyon National Park.

I kept a journal on my trip and on September 7, the day we visited Bryce Canyon, my entry, in all capital letters said, "BEST DAY EVER". I also wrote, again in all capitals, "OH MY GOD—FANTASTIC!!!". I had no other journal entries that even came close to the excitement of this particular day. We awoke and got an early start that day. We headed north on Route 89. When we got back to Route 9, we doubled back toward Zion National Park. We had left the park without taking a picture at the sign the day before so I want-

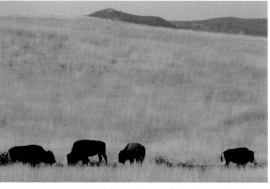

*Buffalo grazing at Zion Mountain Ranch*

ed to go back. We had also passed a herd of buffalo up against the fence right alongside the road. Charlie was in the lead at the time and I couldn't figure out why he didn't stop when we came to the buffalo. There were cars pulled off the side of the road and people everywhere. Damn, I'd missed my opportunity to get a buffalo picture, so we had to go back.

We got our picture at the Zion National Park sign and then stopped at the Zion Mountain Ranch, home of the buffalo herd that we had seen the day before. This morning, the herd was roaming way up in the field, away from the road. We'd missed our chance to see them up front and personal, but we did get to meet a baby buffalo and talk to the rancher about his herd. He explained that they raised the buffalo for their meat. We were surprised when he told us the number of acres, thousands and thousands, that were necessary for a small herd of buffalo to graze.

We left Zion Mountain Ranch and made our way back to Route 89 North. We continued riding north until we got to Route 12 East, which would take us to Bryce Canyon National Park. To our surprise, we had to ride through Red Rock Canyon, lo-

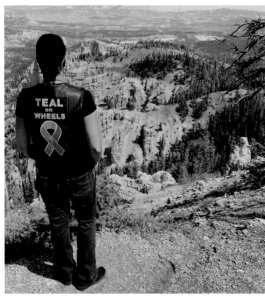

cated nine miles west of Bryce on Scenic Byway 12. Red Rock Canyon is part of the Dixie National Forest. Unique red rock formations and Ponderosa Pines make the canyon a visual delight. Riding through it was just a warm up for what we were about to see when we entered Bryce Canyon National Park. Bryce was my favorite

*Standing at the edge of Bryce Canyon*

of the three National Parks that we visited on our way across southern Utah. As grand and majestic as Zion was, I enjoyed Bryce Canyon more.

We made our way through the entrance and picked up a map of the park. It was a 20-mile drive through the park with scenic viewpoints along the way. Bryce Canyon is a series of large natural amphitheaters with thousands of multi-colored rock pinnacles called "hoodoos." I had never before seen anything in nature that closely resembled the hoodoos. We rode to the farthest point first and then stopped at each scenic viewpoint on our way back to the entrance. There was ample parking at each stop. We got off the bikes and walked to the edge of the canyon taking in the breathtaking views.

The stops were close together and we ran into some of the same park visitors over and over. At one of the scenic viewpoints, a big tour bus was in the small parking area. As we pulled in on our bikes, the passengers were on their way back to the bus. I'm not sure where they were from, but a woman came up to Charlie and me asking, or at least we think she was asking, if she could sit on the bike and get her picture taken. We had a hard time communicating and surmised that she might be French. She was not taking no for an answer when we tried to warn her

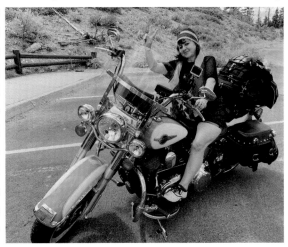

*The woman from the bus*

about the hot exhaust pipes that might burn the exposed skin of her legs. She was wearing shorts. She climbed aboard Charlie's bike first, then mine, all the while instructing her partner to take her picture. She was having a grand time sitting on the two bikes while the bus driver was doing his best to get her back onto the bus. We were glad we only encountered the bus at one of the scenic stops.

The ride was forty miles up and back through the park and the views were absolutely magnificent. I hated to depart when we arrived back at the entrance where we had come in.

We headed back out to Route 12 toward the Grand Staircase-Escalante National Monument, so named for the series of plateaus that descend from Bryce Canyon in the north to the Grand Canyon in the south. It is a United States National Monument originally designated by President Bill Clinton in 1996. It encompassed 1,880,461 acres of protected land in southern Utah. In 2017, the monument's size was reduced by nearly half, to 1,003,863 acres, in a succeeding presidential proclamation. It is the largest national monument managed by the Bureau of Land Management. This area of the continental United States is so rugged and remote that it was the last part of the country to be mapped. We had found a gem and we were riding through it.

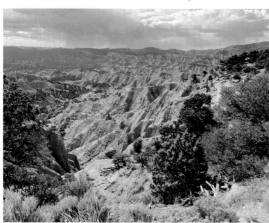

Unlike the surrounding National Parks, Grand Staircase-Escalante had very little traffic, but the most amazing scenery. With each curve in the road, a new vista opened up and they just kept getting better and better. At one point, we came around a bend in the

*A scenic view in Grand Staircase-Escalante N.M.*

road and I pulled to the side. Charlie stopped behind me and asked what was wrong. I said, "Just look at the view. I just had to stop to take it in."

We rode about 120 miles through the National Monument, about half of our total mileage for the day. We were heading to Torrey for the night. It had been a long day of riding and we still had many miles to go. We started at an elevation of 1,343 feet in Kanab and would finish at 6,837 in Torrey, but along the way we reached an elevation of 9,600 feet during our ride. The roads we were

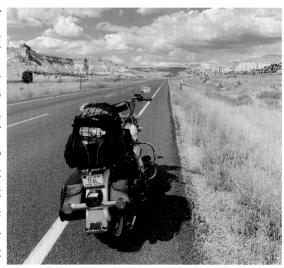

*Route 12...a road to remember*

riding were fantastic—lots of curves and tremendous views. As dusk was approaching, it started to rain. We pulled over to put on our rain gear, hoping we were close to Torrey. I was riding in the lead and as we came down a steep incline, the road curved sharply to the right. As I made the turn, in the last of the day's light with rain gently falling, I came face to face with an 800 plus pound cow standing broadside in the wet roadway. We had been traveling through open range areas for a good part of the afternoon. I had seen cattle off the side of the road, but I wasn't expecting one to be standing broadside in my lane. I hit the brakes hard and got my feet down coming to a stop not very far from the cow. I hoped that Charlie was paying attention behind me. He was, stopping his bike in the outside of the lane next to me. We looked at one another and looked at the cow. I said, "What do we do now?" He replied, "She'll move." We looked to either side of the road where her bovine friends were milling around not paying any attention to us. She was not paying much attention either. It was a little intimidating thinking that if the other cows decided to charge us, we'd be in trouble. Charlie, who as a young boy, worked on a dairy farm, had familiarity with cows. He assured me we were not in any danger. We waited as she slowly moved to the side of the road and we proceeded. Our wildlife spotting that day had included buffalo, cows, turkeys, and prairie dogs. If I had to pick one of those to be in the middle of the road, I would pick the prairie dogs.

It was almost dark when we reached the hotel where we were spending the night. It had been a long day of riding, but it was one of the best days I have ever had on a motorcycle. One of the best parts was that I got to share the day with Charlie.

The next day would be our last day together. We would be riding along Capitol Reef National Park, but we did not have time to explore the area. We were heading for Moab, UT, home of Arches National Park. We had 150 miles to ride before we would even reach the park. We would be spending another night glamping at Under Canvas Moab, adjacent to Arches National Park. We got an early start under threatening skies and made our way across Route 24 East to Route 95 South skirting Capitol Reef National Park on the western side. As we continued on, we crossed the Colorado River and went past Bears Ears National Monument. It was a scenic ride, which would have been better if the sun had been out. Near Blanding we turned north on Route 191 and headed to Moab. We stopped on Route 191 to put on our rain gear just as rain began to fall. We arrived at our destination and decided to unload the bikes at Under Canvas Moab, so we could travel lightly through Arches National Park. The road into this Under Canvas location was not nearly as challenging as the Zion property. By the time we arrived, the sun was out. We unloaded the bikes and headed into town for some lunch.

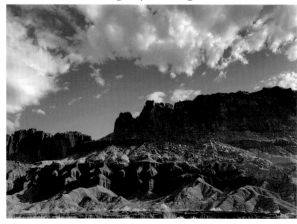

*A view inside Arches N. P.*

After lunch, we headed to Arches National Park. The park is known as the site of more than 2,000 natural sandstone arches, such as the massive, red-hued Delicate Arch in the East. Long, thin Landscape Arch stands in Devils Garden to the North. Other geological formations include Balanced Rock, towering over the desert landscape in the middle of the park. The park contains the highest density of naturally occurring arches in the world. We pulled in and stopped for a picture of the sign at the entrance. Arches National Park, at 76,679 acres was about half the size of Zion at 148,016 acres, and twice the size of Bryce Canyon, 35,835 acres.

We rode through the park taking in the beautiful views of the distant arches. Parking areas at the most popular arches were crowded, so we did not hike in to see any up close. The wind had picked up and it was now blowing pretty hard. We decided to head back to the glampground. When we got back, one of the Under Canvas staff mem-

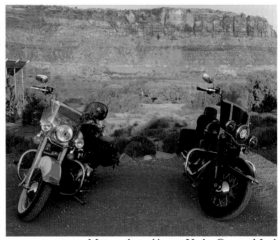

bers told us about a must-do motorcycle ride on Route 128, north of Moab. The route ran parallel to the Colorado River. Charlie decided to go on the ride, but I had had enough riding for the day and decided to stay at the glampground for the rest of the after-

*Motorcycle parking at Under Canvas Moab*

noon. We were not able to ride our bikes right up to our tent site here like we had done at Under Canvas Zion, so we collected our gear that we had left earlier at the reception area and loaded it into one of the available golf carts. We left the bikes parked near the reception tent. The golf cart driver would deliver me and our gear to the tent site and would pick us back up in the morning when we were ready to leave. Tonight would be our last night together. We had enjoyed the last 3 days of riding together, but it would soon be time to part ways.

When Charlie returned from the Route 128 ride, he exclaimed that it was fabulous and I was kind of sad I didn't go with him. I looked at the map and realized that I could go that way in the morning. I could take Route 128 North to Interstate 70 and go east to Colorado. Charlie would take Route 191 North to Route 70 and go west. He would have a long ride back to Salt Lake City the next day and would need to get an early start. He would have to return his rental bike and get to the airport to fly home. I could have a leisurely start in the morning and enjoy the scenic ride north to I-70 East and head into Colorado.

I would get off I-70 in Grand Junction, CO and take Route 50 East across the Rocky Mountains and all the way to Kansas. This would be the next leg of my journey.

*Chapter 15*

# ROLLING THE DICE

**Just four days after leaving the hospital** from my extended stay for the collapsed lung, I resumed my treatments. Every week, I left my home on Swan's Island and traveled to Bar Harbor for my chemotherapy session. Charlie took me sometimes, a couple times I drove myself, and several times, one of my friends on Swan's Island drove me. My friend Tom took me once and another time my friend Carolyn was my driver. It was hard for Charlie to miss a full day of work each week, so when someone offered to drive me, I usually accepted. I was grateful for the help.

Having chemo every seven days presented a lot of challenges. It took about 14 weeks to get to my tenth chemo treatment. My hospitalization for the collapsed lung delayed treatment by two weeks, then I had some issues with my blood counts—my white blood cell count, my platelet count, and my red blood cell count at times were all too low. All of these things interfered with getting my treatment on time.

When I left my tenth round of chemo, my nurse Melanie asked me the same question she asked me every week, "Do you have any tingling or numbness in your hands or feet?" I told her I had the slightest bit of tingling in my feet. She told me to make sure I told my oncologist, Dr. Brooks, about it the following Thursday when I saw him. One of the chemo drugs I was getting, Taxol, was known to cause peripheral neuropathy, damage to the nerves in the extremities—the hands and feet. The "pins and needles" feeling was only a slight sensation affecting both feet on Friday when I reported it to Melanie. By the next day, my feet felt like they were on fire. I could barely walk the eight steps from my bedroom to my bathroom. I could not put on socks or shoes. In bed, I could not even pull a sheet up over my feet. It was too painful. I had never experienced anything like this before. I saw Dr. Brooks the following week and he told me the neuropathy was from the Taxol. He said it could get worse and it could be permanent. I couldn't imagine how it could get any worse than it already was. He gave me a break from my chemo and said we would reassess my condition the following week. We agreed that if I had great improvement during my week off chemo, I would resume treatment the following week and have my eleventh round of the eighteen chemo sessions I was scheduled to have. My neuropathy did not improve, or if it did, it was so slight that it was not noticeable to me. I struggled all week about whether to continue chemo or stop. I kept hearing Dr. Brooks' voice in my head saying the neuropathy could get worse and it could be permanent. I was consumed with trying to make a very difficult decision. In the morning, Charlie would leave for work and I would say, I'm quitting chemo. He'd come home for lunch and I would say, I'm going back on Thursday for more chemo. I flip-flopped trying to make my decision. I thought my best chance for long-term survival was to finish the course of treatment that my two GYN oncologists, Dr. Small and Dr. Wright, had recommended. After all, they were the experts on ovarian cancer. On

Wednesday, the day before my next chemo session, my oncology nurse Joyce called me. She asked me if I was coming in for my chemo the next day. I was put on the spot and needed an answer. I'd given this hours and hours of thought, yet I still didn't know for sure what the right thing to do was. Pressed for an answer, I blurted out, "I'm quitting chemo." I just couldn't risk the neuropathy getting any worse and there was no way I could take a chance on it being permanent. There, I had made my decision. I was rolling the dice for quality of life—even if it came at the cost of less quantity of life. Joyce did not try to change my mind, and for that I was grateful.

# Chapter 16

# ELVIS

**I had no particular itinerary** for my Teal on Wheels ride across the country—just a starting point, Coos Bay, Oregon and a stopping point, Swan's Island, Maine. My only other commitments were being in Salt Lake City, Utah to meet Charlie, when he arrived, and being in Royersford, Pennsylvania, for a fundraiser my high school friends had planned to help me raise money for my cause. The rest of my time was wide open, I could go wherever I wanted and explore this awe-inspiring country I call home.

I traveled with a copy of the 2019 Harley Owners Group Touring Handbook, an eight by ten and a half inch, 139-page book. This handbook included the location of all the Harley dealers in the country, important information in case I had any trouble with the bike along the way, or just needed an oil change, which I did. The guide, more importantly, included maps of all 50 states and highlighted, in yellow, the most scenic motorcycle routes in each state. I had no intention of riding mile after mile on the interstates and highways. That was not my idea of fun. The highlighted routes, included in the handbook, were the dream of any adventurous motorcycle rider—roads off the beaten path with long sweeping curves and magnificent scenery. They were certainly not the shortest or quickest routes to get from point A to point B, but I was on a bucket list trip and wanted to see the country, so this travel guide quickly became invaluable to me. I did not realize at the beginning of my trip how important this collection of maps would be. Each morning it was one of the last things I loaded back onto my bike. I carefully folded it in half and tucked it under the cargo net that I stretched over the bag that rode on my passenger seat behind me. That way I could easily find it if I needed it during the day, and I wouldn't have to rifle through my saddlebags looking for it. I consulted the maps every night before I went to sleep to get a sense of where the next day's riding would take me.

When I reached Clarksville, Arkansas, I decided to take a rest day after 18 straight days of riding. I had not intended to ride that many days in a row. My original plan at the start of the trip was to incorporate one rest day into each week of riding, but my excitement at the start of the trip was so great that I just kept riding. By the time I reached Clarksville, Arkansas I was tired and needed to rest, so I parked the bike and stayed at the same hotel for two nights. I walked down the hill both nights from the Quality Inn I was staying at to eat at El Molcajete, a great little Mexican restaurant. On my first night at El Molcajete, I told the cashier about my Teal on Wheels trip and gave her one of my ovarian cancer symptom cards. We chatted for a short while and in the end, she charged me only for the two beers I had and gave me my meal for free. This happened quite frequently as I traveled across the country. It made me feel like there were indeed many kind and caring people in the world.

My need for rest, both physically and mentally, was obvious to me by the time I reached Clarksville. The hot days were taking a toll on me—riding in all my motorcycle gear was not like traveling by car where you have your drink in the cup holder and you are wearing shorts and flip flops. Traveling by motorcycle is very different, especially when you are dressing for safety. Helmet, boots, jacket are all very hot. I only stopped for something to drink when I stopped for gas for the bike, on most days that was not enough. I was becoming dehydrated and at first I did not realize it. I'm sure my nightly beers didn't help this either. My much needed two day rest in Clarksville gave me plenty of time to plan the next part of my journey. I consulted my touring guide and flipped back and forth from the Arkansas map on page 9 to the Tennessee map on page 22. I realized I was a mere 200 miles west of Memphis, Tennessee. Beale Street, home of the blues, and Graceland, home of Elvis were there. I just had to go to Memphis. Up to this point in the trip, I had pretty much stayed away from large cities, except for Salt Lake City in Utah, so Memphis would present something new and different for me. I was more than halfway across the country, but the excitement of the trip had not faded. At the start of the trip, I thought it might—thought that maybe I would have to face reality, that maybe I had bitten off more than I could chew attempting a ride of this magnitude. But, I was still just as excited as I was on day one of the trip.

I looked forward to crossing the mighty Mississippi River- er and arriving in Memphis. I was traveling east on I-40 in six lanes of traffic as I approached the Hernando de Soto Bridge that would take me across the river. As a young school girl, I remember learning about

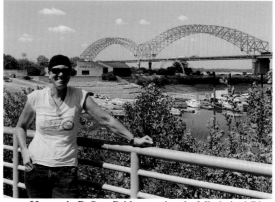

*Hernando DeSoto Bridge crossing the Mississippi River*

the Mississippi River and now here I was riding my motorcycle across it. I have to admit, it was not as impressive as I thought it would be. I somehow imagined the river would be bigger, but nevertheless, crossing the Mississippi meant my journey was moving eastward.

My first stop was the Memphis Visitor's Center. I knew nothing about navigating around Memphis. I would need to get my bearings. It was another sweltering day in the South and you'd think by now I would have grown accustomed to the heat, but I had not. Each day seemed hotter than the day before, but the excitement of yet another adventure kept me going.

At the Visitor's Center, I met a fellow rider who had left Texas in the wee hours of the morning and was headed to visit family in Missouri. He seemed like a good ole boy with an American flag proudly flying off the back of his big full dresser Harley-Davidson, a bike much bigger than mine and meant to ride long distances. He asked me to take a couple of pictures of him. I asked the same in return.

Inside the Visitor's Center stood a huge bronze statue of Elvis Presley with a guitar. No doubt, I had reached Memphis. A stop here was every music lover's dream. I wanted to visit Beale Street, where so many musicians had gotten their start, but that would have to wait. First, I needed to secure a room for the night—a place to cool off for a spell before beginning my exploration of the city. A woman working behind the counter helped me find a room by offering me a coupon book and suggested I stay at the Day's Inn—a good spot within walking distance to Graceland. It sounded good to me, so Day's Inn Memphis was my next destination.

Thank goodness for my GPS. I plugged in the address of the Day's Inn and wound along the waterfront and back onto the highway. I traveled a few more miles before going past the huge Graceland complex. I spotted my hotel just up the road. I had not been steered wrong—it was a great location. I pulled in, shut off my bike's engine, and was immediately greeted by the sounds of Elvis' Blue Suede Shoes blasting from a set of outdoor speakers. I wondered to myself, will this music be playing all night? How will I ever get any sleep here? I approached the reception desk and produced the coupon for the discounted rate—$94 for the night. Before moving my bike down the hill to the outside entrance to my room, I peaked into a courtyard behind the office and to my surprise there was a guitar shaped swimming pool. It was filled with senior citizens of all shapes and sizes. I figured all of them had probably visited Graceland earlier in the day and were now cooling off from the oppressive heat. I decided against going swimming to cool off and retreated to my room where I cranked up the air conditioning hoping for some relief.

I was only a block away from Graceland and decided to visit that afternoon. I changed out of my riding clothes and put on a tank top, a skirt and some flip flops and down the sidewalk I strolled toward Graceland. I was expecting a fairly substantial house to tour—but the whole Elvis experience was much more than I had imagined. On the opposite side of the highway from Graceland stood a whole complex dedicated to everything Elvis—multiple buildings housing Elvis' collections of cars, boats, motorcycles, and even racing golf carts. Elvis' gold records, his costumes, and even some of his movies were playing. Photos and memorabilia from his time in the Army were well preserved and on display. You could even tour two of Elvis' personal airplanes.

I purchased the upgraded ticket that gave me access not only to Graceland, but to all of the rest, too. After all, I was at Graceland and I wanted to see it all! The experience started with a short movie about Elvis' life. After that we were ushered to a cattle shoot outside where we waited in line for a tour bus to take us across the highway to Elvis' estate. While waiting in line, we were each given a headset and an iPad that contained a self-guided tour of Graceland. I saw women waiting in line for the bus that were carrying bouquets of red roses. I assumed they would place them on Elvis' grave. I thought about my mom—she would have done that if she had ever gotten the chance to visit Graceland. She was the one who introduced me to music—Elvis, the Beatles, and anything Rock n' Roll were among her favorites.

We hurried onto the bus, which took us a few hundred yards out of the complex and across the highway to Graceland. I could have easily walked there, but you had to arrive on the bus I was told. Just a minute later we were at the front door of Graceland, but we had to wait to get inside. We were told there would be a slight delay before our group could enter. We were asked to step

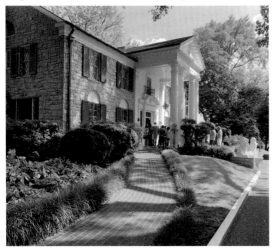

*GRACELAND - home of Elvis Presley*

away from the front entrance. A wedding party soon made an appearance and took center stage in front of the mansion—a perfect backdrop for wedding party photos of a Memphis wedding. I wondered how much it had cost them to do this. Did they get married by an Elvis-like preacher? Would their marriage be like Elvis and Priscilla? I hoped not. Finally the photographer snapped his last image and it was our turn to walk up the steps and enter Graceland.

I listened intently to the stories on my iPad device as I moved from room to room with my group of Elvis devotees. The flashy furnishings that adorned each room, unchanged since the 1970s, brought to life what Elvis, his family, and his entourage did inside these walls and on the grounds of Graceland. I could picture it just as if it was happening right before my eyes.

Toward the end of the tour, we were funneled out into a meditation garden behind the estate. This was the highlight of the tour, what everyone wanted to see—Elvis' final resting place. It was a peaceful water fountain display with the graves of Elvis and his family members stretching out like rays of the sun from the center of the circle. Surrounded by his parents, Gladys and Vernon Presley's memorial markers, Elvis' grave site was adorned with red roses, small stuffed animals, and notes of adoration left by his many fans who visit Graceland every day. Elvis' death, at the age of 42, left a huge hole in the music world. I was only 17 years old when Elvis Presley's life tragically ended—not old enough to be a fan in my own right, but old enough to remember him and understand the impact he had on early Rock n' Roll. That day, August 16, 1977, the music world lost a legend.

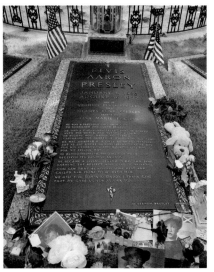

*Elvis Presley's gravesite*

*Chapter 17*

# THE BRAZILIANS

**Memphis had so much to see and do.** It wasn't all about Elvis and Graceland. There was so much more. I wanted to see Beale Street—American's most iconic street, Home of the Blues. I was too scared to go to Beale Street by myself after dark. I imagined it might be full of all kinds of seedy characters and was unsure how safe a visit at night would be. I definitely didn't want to ride my bike there after dark, so I decided to visit in the early morning hours.

I found a parking lot adjacent to the entrance to Beale Street. It was empty when I arrived, but I'm sure it had been filled to capacity the night before. As I walked toward the start of Beale Street, I passed by a small police station and thought to myself how appropriate that seemed—a police station next to the city's largest partying place. In the early morning hours,

Beale Street seemed deserted. I was greeted by an overhead structure that spanned the width of the street welcoming me. As I walked along the sidewalk, I felt like I was in sensory overload. Bars, restaurants, and storefronts, brightly painted, lined both sides of the street for blocks. A variety of classic music genres like blues, jazz, Rock 'n' Roll, and gospel were celebrated here. Brass musical notes with names of early musicians were embedded in the concrete sidewalk, just like I thought Hollywood's Walk of Fame might look, only older and dingier—not as brightly polished. Haunts named after some of the greats Jerry Lee Lewis' Cafe and Honky Tonk and B.B. King's Blues Club to name a couple. And then there were the food joints, many featuring Memphis-style BBQ.

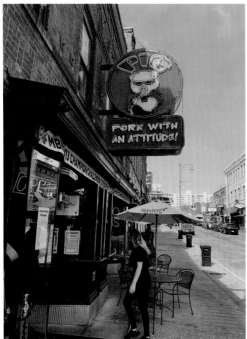

*Pork with an Attitude BBQ Joint*

As I strolled along, I was wishing I had come here the night before to experience the people, the music, the beer and food—the whole Beale Street atmosphere. But maybe it was best that I hadn't.

After taking it all in, I left Beale Street and made my way back to the parking lot where I had parked my motorcycle. It was early in the day, but I knew it was going to be another hot day in the South. I wound my way through some less exciting parts of Memphis trying to find another historic attraction that I was looking for—the Lorraine Motel, the place where Martin Luther King, Jr. was assassinated on April 4, 1968. I was 8 years old at the time of King's death and knew nothing of the civil rights movement growing up in rural Pennsylvania. King, a Christian minister and activist was the most visible spokesperson for the civil rights movement from 1955 until his assassination. Adjacent to the Lorraine Motel, the National Civil Rights

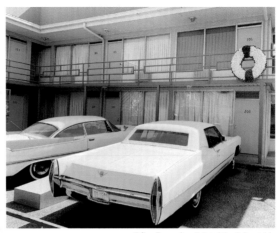

*The Lorraine Motel in Memphis*

Museum was built. It opened to the public on September 28, 1991. The Lorraine Motel, located at 450 Mulberry Street in Memphis, maintains the original look of 1968. A large memorial wreath hangs from the second floor balcony outside Room 306, where King was standing at the time of his assassination. Parked just below Room 306 are two cars, a white 1959 Dodge Royal with lime green fins and a white 1968 Cadillac. The scene seems to be suspended in time.

A group of about a dozen men were visiting the site at the same time I was. I wasn't sure of their nationality, but they were speaking a foreign language. The mood was somber, so I did not attempt to engage in conversation as I read the various kiosks filled with information about this historic event. I moved beyond the Lorraine Motel to the entrance to the National Civil Rights Museum. I gave a tug on the door, but it did not open. I tugged again, but still nothing. I looked on the door where the hours were posted and to my dismay the Museum was closed on Tuesdays and here it was Tuesday morning. I was disappointed and thought for a moment about whether or not I could spend another night in Memphis. I decided I could not. As I turned to leave, I spoke to the men and said, "The Museum is closed today. It's closed on Tuesdays." I was not sure if they understood me. I made my way to my bike and headed out of Memphis.

My time spent in Memphis was hot and humid and I was hoping if I got out of the city I would find some cooler riding. I was growing tired of all of the hot days—temperatures in the 90s and over 100 degrees on some days. I was 20 days into the ride and I had not had any cool weather riding since my first day heading down to California. The heat was taking its toll on me. I was becoming more dehydrated each day. I was having a difficult time taking in enough fluids while riding. Not only was I losing fluids, I was losing weight, too. I found it very challenging to eat during the day. I started to become concerned about my health.

As I left Memphis, I was looking for the Natchez Trace Parkway. The Parkway is a 444-mile recreational road and scenic drive through three states, starting in Natchez, Mississippi, through parts of Alabama, and ending in Nashville, Tennessee. I thought I could enter the Parkway at one of the many access points along the route and that I would find one not too far from Memphis. I was wrong about that.

I continued eastward, or what I thought was eastward looking for the Parkway. I finally stopped at a small mini-mart gas station. I got off my bike, grabbed my Harley touring guide and went inside to take advantage of the air conditioning at a small eatery located inside the building. I grabbed a couple bottles of water, sat down, and opened my map book. Two elderly gentlemen were sitting nearby. One asked, "Where you going?" I replied that I was looking for the Natchez Trace Parkway. He told me to continue east on the road I was on until I got to Alabama. I asked him if I was still in Tennessee and he informed me that I was now in Mississippi. WHAT? I had been looking for cooler weather, but had traveled further south. I was now in Mississippi and heading toward Alabama. He continued on with his directions telling me I would see a big green sign about 30 miles down the road and that would be the welcome to Alabama sign and that the Natchez Trace Parkway entrance would be a little way beyond that. I thanked him and made my way out to my bike. I opened one of the bottles of water, leaned forward, and dumped it on my head to cool off. I put my helmet on, climbed aboard my bike and was on my way again.

I finally found the entrance to the Natchez Trace Parkway and it was well worth the little jaunt south to get there. The riding on the Parkway was delightful with little traffic. I was also able to add two more states, Mississippi and Alabama, to my list of states travelled through during my journey.

In my trip journal for that day, I wrote, "HOT AS HELL!!!" I stopped after crossing the Tennessee River and made a short video on my iPhone about how hot it was that day. I continued on making my way to Columbia, TN for the night after riding 238 miles that day.

I was finally on the eastern side of Tennessee and would be traveling through the Great Smoky Mountains soon. I had been looking forward to getting up into the mountains hoping for cooler weather and was especially excited about riding on the Blue Ridge Parkway. The Blue Ridge Parkway is a National Parkway and designated as an All-American Road noted for its scenic beauty. The Parkway, which is America's longest linear park, runs for 469 miles through 29 Virginia and North Carolina counties, linking the Great Smoky Mountains National Park to Shenandoah National Park. I wouldn't ride the whole 469 miles, but I would ride part of the way on the Parkway.

I stayed in Pigeon Forge that night—home of Dollywood, Dolly Parton's amusement park. I somehow pictured Dollywood to be the only attraction in Pigeon Forge, nestled in a tiny rural town off the beaten path. It was nothing like I imagined at all. Pigeon Forge is a vacation mecca with a highway running right through the center of the city. Amusements parks and museums, country music venues and dinner theaters, shopping outlets, restaurants and bars all lined the main drag. The commercial district was bustling with activity and attractions.

When I got up the next morning, I did not feel well, but I was excited to be heading into the Great Smoky Mountains National Park. It took me forever to get ready and load up my motorcycle. I had a nagging feeling that I should just stay at the hotel for another night, but I also wanted to continue on. Eventually I was ready to go and my first stop was a gas station and convenience store not far from my hotel. Just like the start of every day, I topped off my gas tank and grabbed a few bottles of Gatorade, water, and some snacks. As I was storing my supplies on my bike, I was overcome with a feeling that something was not right. I couldn't shake the feeling. I felt weak and tired and was concerned about getting on the bike and riding. I was 23 days into the trip and had only taken one rest day just five days earlier in Clarksville, Arkansas. I felt like I needed to push on, so I got on the road and started down US 441 heading south towards Gatlinburg about 8 miles away. Another 10 miles after that and I would be at the park entrance. By the time I got to Gatlinburg, a quaint mountain town, traffic was bumper to bumper. It was not only full of vehicles, but the sidewalks were overflowing with tourists. It was stop and go and I just wanted to get to the far side of the town. Finally, the traffic started moving again and it was not

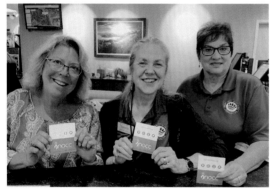

*Handing out my symptom cards*

long before I reached the entrance to the National Park. Just inside the entrance, I stopped at the Visitor's Center. There I met three of the nicest volunteers at the counter. I told them all about my trip and gave each one of them an ovarian cancer symptom card. I got a map of the park and was on my way.

I started through the park and was heading up to the highest point, Clingmans Dome. I didn't get very far when I was overcome by dizziness. I wasn't sure what was happening to me, but I knew I needed to stop riding immediately. As soon as I could safely pull over, I did. I got off the bike and sat down on the curb of the small parking area I had entered. I wasn't sure what to do. I went back to my bike and got a bottle of Gatorade and some pretzels. I was pretty sure I was suffering from dehydration from the last three weeks of riding in oppressive heat. I drank as much as I could and tried to come up with a plan. I didn't have a cell phone signal, so I couldn't call for help. I decided to make a short video on my phone detailing where I was and what was happening to me. I thought if I had an accident on the bike the video would let people know what had happened to me. After a while of just sitting, I decided to see if I could safely ride. I got back on my bike and started it up. I decided I would not go to Clingmans Dome as I had originally planned to do, but instead I would ride across the mountain and into North Carolina to try and find some medical help. As I climbed higher and higher in elevation to get across the mountains, I found myself riding inside some low lying clouds. At first I thought it was fog, but then realized I was riding inside of a cloud. The cool, damp air felt good to me, but the lack of visibility, like riding in a dense fog, was concerning. I needed all my senses and I didn't have them. I passed the turn to Clingmans Dome, but didn't take it. I wanted to be off this mountain as quickly as possible and that was not going to be the way. I stopped at a scenic overlook, but couldn't see a thing. I went into the bathroom. The inside of the stall door had a big warning sign, "Watch Out for Elk". I could barely see 10 feet in front of me riding inside the clouds, I was feeling awful, and now I had to watch out for elk, too. I made it off the mountain and arrived in Cherokee, NC. I found a hotel and asked for a room. It was too early to check-in, but I told the desk clerk that I was having medical issues and needed to be off my bike. I asked her if there was a medical clinic in the town and she gave me the number. I was hoping that I could get some IV fluids. I knew that would fix me right up. I called the number once I got to my room. I was told that the clinic in town only took care of tribal members, Native Americans. They could not help me. They suggested I call the local hospital and gave me the number. I called, explained my situation, that I was hoping to get some IV fluids. I was told I would have to go through the ER. I was not willing to go through all of that, so I put my shoes on and walked to the nearest convenience store and bought more Gatorade and more water. I also got a sandwich to eat. It was barely 10am and I had only ridden 50 miles, but I felt like I had been on the road all day. I went back to my room and proceeded to drink and drink and drink, all day and all night.

When I woke up the next morning, the sun was shining brightly and it was a new day. I felt much better. I loaded up my bike, thanked the desk clerk, who was the same woman from the day before who let me check-in early, turned my bike around and headed back into the Great Smoky Mountains National Park. I wanted to see what I had missed the day before.

I was not disappointed. I rode to Clingmans Dome. At 6,643 feet, it is the highest point in the Park. The "Dome" refers to the mountaintop, not the man-made observation tower that is located there. On clear days, like that day, you could enjoy a 100 mile view in every direction.

I left the Clingmans Dome parking area and traveled back the seven miles to the main road to continue on my way. I stopped at another scenic area with a large parking lot. It was filled with cars and campers. I spotted a large group of motorcycles parked there. After taking some pictures and enjoying the view, I head-

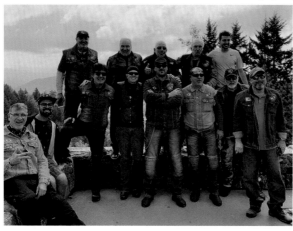

*Me and the Condores no Asfalto from São Paulo, Brazil*

ed back across the parking lot towards my bike. I heard someone shouting, "Wait, wait." I turned to see a man waving at me and calling out to me. I walked back towards him. He said, "I know you." I did not recognize him. He spoke with a heavy accent that I could not recognize. He insisted that he knew me and tried to explain in his broken English that we had met before at the museum. Again, I told him I did not know him. Then he said, "At the museum in Memphis." I remembered, he was part of the group of men that were visiting the National Civil Rights Museum the day it was closed. He motioned me to come and meet his friends. We walked over to the group and he began to tell them who I was. This time they were all dressed in motorcycle riding clothes. When I saw them in Memphis, they were riding in several big black SUVs, the kind government officials ride around in. There was a younger man with them who spoke good English. I quickly learned that they were from Brazil. They were on a guided motorcycle tour and had started in New Orleans. I asked if I could get a picture with all of them and it was like herding cats, me speaking in English, them not sure what I wanted them to do. Finally, with the help of lots of hand gesturing, I got them all lined up and convinced a passerby to take a group photo with my cell phone. We said our goodbyes and I headed back to my bike. Again, someone called out to me, "Wait!" I stopped, looked back and one of the men came hurrying across the parking lot and presented me with a gift. It was a special neckerchief wrapped in plastic that they had made for this trip. It featured a cartoon-like Condor sitting on a motorcycle with a helmet and googles on. It featured a US flag and a Brazilian flag. Their riding group was called Condores no Asfalto, which translates to Condors of the Asphalt. I graciously accepted the gift and we finally parted ways.

I headed down off the mountains and found my way onto the Blue Ridge Parkway. My next stop was Maggie Valley, North Carolina, where I planned to visit Dale Walksler's Wheels Through Time Motorcycle Museum. I made a couple of stops at scenic overlooks on the parkway and at my last stop, as I was putting on my helmet and getting on my bike, I heard the loud rumble of engines, lots of engines, getting closer. I turned to look back at the entrance of the turnout and here came my new friends, the Brazilians. They pulled in and backed their bikes into the parking spots at the edge of the paved area. We immediately started laughing when we saw one another. I asked them if they were following me. Then, I asked where they were heading next and one of them said, "Wheels Through Time." I told them that's where

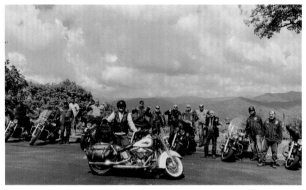

I was heading. They were going to stop for lunch first and asked me to join them. I declined their offer. Having lunch with more than a dozen Brazilian motorcycle riding men seemed like it would be an all day affair. We took some pictures of us and our bikes and I was on my way. I had a feeling I might see them again at the Motorcycle Museum, but I was there and gone before they arrived.

*Meeting up with the Brazilians again*

It seemed funny to me that I would cross paths with the Brazilians three times in four days. I hope they enjoyed their trip to the United States. I know I enjoyed running into them over and over again.

*Chapter 18*

# LOOKING FOR QUALITY OF LIFE

**Shortly after stopping chemo** in September 2016, I started a drug called Letrozole, also known as Femara. Women with hormone receptor positive cancer, like some ovarian cancer patients including me, and many breast cancer patients, are treated with Letrozole or other aromatase inhibitor drugs. Aromatase inhibitors stop the production of estrogen in postmenopausal women. This means that less estrogen is available to stimulate the growth of hormone receptor positive cancer cells. In a really simplified explanation, taking this drug would hopefully cut off the "food supply" to my cancer.

The Letrozole worked really great for me—it doesn't work for all women. It stabilized my remaining cancer and eventually reduced my cancer load. I was on it for nearly four years, stopping it in July 2020. In the summer of 2020, I was not doing well and I was sick of the side effects of the Letrozole. The most serious side effects of the drug involved the bones: fractures, decreased bone density, and osteoporosis. I went from having great bone density when I started the drug to osteopenia, low bone density, very quickly. I did not lose enough bone density to be diagnosed with osteoporosis, but I came close. I had constant joint pain, muscle pain, hot flashes, weakness, insomnia, and increased cholesterol—all side effects of Letrozole. I'm not sure which was worse, the chemo or the Letrozole. I think the Letrozole, but maybe because I was on it for so long. When I first started the drug, the bone pain was in my lower back and my lower legs. I remember sweeping my kitchen floor one day and when I leaned down with the dust pan and dust brush, I fell onto the floor. I lay there in a pile of dog fur in the middle of my kitchen floor. I had no idea what was happening to me. I had been in great physical shape prior to my cancer diagnosis. I could easily lift a fifty pound bag of dog food or a big bag of mulch for my flowerbed. Now I was weak and fragile. I just wanted the old me back.

After about six months on the Letrozole, I reached out to Dr. David Gershenson at MD Anderson Cancer Center in Houston, Texas. Dr. Gershenson is known as the guru of low grade serous ovarian cancer. He was the lead researcher on Letrozole and low grade cancer patients. I was on this drug because of him. I was amazed when he emailed me back in less than 24 hours with a response to my inquiry about the side effects of the drug. I called them debilitating. He suggested a break of two weeks to see if my condition improved. He was not familiar with patients claiming the degree of pain I was experiencing. I stopped the Letrozole and greatly improved by the end of the two week period. It was the only treatment available to me at the time, so I resumed it after my break. I continued on it until the summer of 2020. I took several two week breaks throughout that time, each time feeling better off the drug. In July 2020, I was feeling rather poorly. I'd had a couple of serious bowel obstructions, the second one landing me in the hospital and lasting nearly a week. I felt like my health was going downhill. I had been given a 5-year prognosis at Dana Farber when I was first diagnosed. I had just passed the four year mark. I was afraid my life might be nearing the end. I just wanted to feel better again for a while, so I stopped taking the Letrozole. This time, two weeks passed, then four weeks. I was beginning to improve. I knew the responsible thing to do was resume the drug, but I just couldn't do it. I was feeling empowered, as if I was taking control of my life back, even if it was the wrong thing to do. I had an oncology appointment with Dr. Brooks and told him I had stopped the Letrozole. At that point, it had been three months. He talked me into trying another one of the aromatase inhibitor drugs, Exemestane. I got the prescription filled at my local pharmacy, but instead of taking the pills, I put it in my cupboard. I was being a defiant patient and I didn't care. I could not bring myself to start the new drug. I was once again rolling the dice in search of better quality of life, just like I had done when I quit my chemo. I've often said I don't care how long I live, only how well I live. And I was feeling better than I had felt in a long time.

In January 2021, seven months after stopping the Letrozole, I had a CT scan of the chest, abdomen, and pelvic area. I don't normally get nervous about my scans, but in this particular case I was. I knew if my cancer had grown significantly during the period that I had not been taking the Letrozole or the Exemestane, that I would have no one to blame but myself. I had gone against the advice of my medical team by stopping my only treatment option. The results of my scan came back. For the first time in 4 years and 9 months, I was declared NED—no evidence of disease. This was great news! But I also know that stage IV ovarian cancer does not just go away—it is lurking somewhere and will rear its ugly head at some point in the future. For now though, I am NED and that's a great thing to be able to say after all this time.

My health issues are a long way from over, but at least my cancer is stable for now. I continue to have multiple bowel obstructions each year, which means multiple hospitalizations. I am on a special diet, a low fiber diet, which means no fruits, no vegetables, no beans, nuts or seeds—the opposite of what every doctor tells you to eat. This diet helps to reduce the number of obstructions that I have. I'm also receiving IV iron infusions on a regular basis due to my inability to absorb enough iron from my diet. I have been diagnosed with cardiac issues—perhaps the long term use of the Letrozole was a contributing factor, but I will never know for sure. There have been studies done that support this theory. In January 2019, I was diagnosed with atrial fibrillation, or A Fib for short. It is an irregular heart rhythm in the atrial chambers of the heart. An atrial septal aneurysm was found in January 2021 and I started on Xarelto, a blood thinner at that time. In March of 2021, a patent foramen ovale, a hole between the right and left atrial chambers was discovered. At the same time, a moderately leaking tricuspid valve was revealed. The tricuspid valve controls blood flow from the right atrial chamber to the right ventricle chambers. When the tricuspid valve does not close tightly enough, it allows blood to flow backward into the right upper heart chamber when the ventricle chamber contracts.

In November 2020, I had a very scary event on the deck of the ferry going home. I had just returned from a 220 mile ride on my motorcycle when I suffered an episode that was very much like a TIA, transient ischemic attack, or mini stroke. This was my second similar event and it could have ended very badly if I had experienced it while I was on my motorcycle.

I feel like I went from being a very fit woman at age 56 when my cancer was diagnosed and over the last five years I have turned into an old woman. No matter how hard I try, I cannot find my way back to my former good health. It is beyond frustrating. My saving grace is my mental health. I have always felt that my mental health was good, even great. A cancer journey like mine does not just affect your body, it affects your mind, too.

Riding my motorcycle is my mental health therapy. When I am on my bike rolling down the road, I do not think of myself as being sick. There's nothing I love more than riding. One day, while riding down a highway, I penned a letter in my head to my cancer. When I got to my hotel for the night I got out my iPad and made the letter more permanent. It started…Dear Cancer, and I shared with my cancer all of the ways it had negatively affected my life. The letter ended with…you may win the war, but today I won the battle. On that day, as I was riding along enjoying the scenery, I was in charge. I did not feel sick. Cancer was not controlling my life. On that day, on my Harley, I was in charge of my own destiny—even if only for a short while.

## Chapter 19

# VIRGINIA CREW

**About a year before I left on my cross country ride,** I met the most amazing group of motorcycle riders from Virginia. The tale of how we met in Rockland, Maine is a fun story. I never thought I would see any of them again, but when they heard about my Teal on Wheels ride, they insisted I visit with them when I got to Virginia. I had only spent a short time with them in Maine, but they were the kind of people you felt like you had known for years. The story of how we met needs to be shared.

In August of 2018, I found myself heading to Rockland, Maine on my 2014 Harley-Davidson Softail Deluxe. It looked like a couple of nice weather days ahead, so I decided to ride my bike the 180 miles down and back from my home on Swan's Island. When I arrived at my hotel I noticed several Harley-Davidson motorcycles, full dressers, the kind of motorcycles built for long distance riding. They were lined up in the parking lot behind the hotel. The bikes were all sporting Virginia license plates. I pulled up to the group of bikes, but then decided to park in the lot on the front side of the hotel. I was hoping to get a room where I would be able to see my bike from my window.

I was in Rockland for several important back-to-back meetings. At the time, I was serving on the Board of Trustees for the non-profit organization, Island Institute. One of the meetings on my schedule was on the offshore island of North Haven and the other one was at Island Institute's office in Rockland, a few blocks from the hotel. I was particularly excited about the first meeting, an all-day trustee event on North Haven, an island about 12 miles off the coast. I would be taking a ferry boat ride, along with other trustees and Island Institute staff to get to the island. My hotel was located directly across the road from the ferry terminal, so it would be a short walk to where the ferry would be loading the next morning.

I must say I am most comfortable in riding jeans, boots and a T-shirt, but when I woke up to get ready to go to North Haven the following morning I knew I couldn't dress like that. Instead, I had packed a dress and a pair of stylish sandals that would be my outfit for the day. The dress, mostly pink in color, was NOT my color, but it was comfortable and I thought it looked good on me. I got showered and dressed and headed down for the complimentary breakfast in the lobby area of the hotel before heading over to board the ferry. Summer is the tourist season in Maine and by the time I got downstairs, the breakfast area was packed with hungry vacationers. It turned out the Annual Lobster Festival was going on in town and it was the busiest week of the summer. The hotel was filled to capacity. I made my way over to one of the waffle makers, bumping into other hotel guests who were all starting their days, too. I wanted a waffle, but the line for the waffle maker was too long, so I opted for some scrambled eggs. I spotted a large man, sporting a big white beard, and wearing a black leather motorcycle vest on top of what I obviously recognized as riding attire. As soon as the opportunity presented itself, I struck up a conversation with him about motorcycles and riding. We exchanged pleasantries and I finished getting some food. I turned to look for a place to sit down and eat, but every table was already occupied. It seemed like there was no empty spot for a single woman in a pink dress. Then I spotted them—the rest of the white bearded man's motorcycle crew. They were sitting at one of those higher tables and there were a couple of empty seats. The bearded man, who had introduced himself as Jim, had not gotten there yet, but I assumed they were part of his group. I wandered over and asked if I could join them. They were big men, but not as big as Jim, but still the kind of men you wouldn't mess around with. They were decked out in Harley gear from head to toe—no mistaking them for anything but motorcycle riders. One of them responded to my request to join them indicating it would be fine. I felt sure they were wondering who the hell is this woman and why did she pick our table. I pulled out a chair and climbed up to the big table with my plate of scrambled eggs. Their plates were overflowing with food—big eaters I thought, but I would have thought that anyway even if I hadn't seen what they were eating. I broke the ice by telling them I had been talking to their friend Jim over by the waffle maker. I asked if the bikes parked out back of the hotel were their bikes and added, "I ride, too. My bike is parked out front." That's all it took. We started chatting about motorcycles and riding. They were in Maine for vacation. They'd ridden up from Virginia. They were hard core, long distance riders. They had been to Acadia National Park riding earlier in the week, and had taken the ferry over to Vinalhaven, another island off the coast from Rockland. On this day, they were planning to stay in town and eat lobsters. I told them I was headed on the ferry to North Haven. We parted ways after I finished my breakfast. They were some good ole boys and I enjoyed talking with them.

Before making my way over to the ferry terminal, I walked around behind the hotel and put one of my business cards on one of their bikes. I realized we had not exchanged information and I wanted them to be able to contact me if they ever wanted to.

Then I was off for a full day of networking, friendship, and good food. It was a long, enjoyable day and evening and I returned after dark on a lobster-type boat that served as a passenger ferry. It was raining pretty hard on the ocean crossing from North Haven back to Rockland. It was a short walk in the pouring rain from the pier where we landed back to the hotel. I must have looked like a drowned rat by the time I walked into the hotel lobby. I had not planned on any rain that day and only had a light jacket, but no umbrella. I strolled into the lobby and heard this loud roar of voices calling my name, "DONNA!" I looked over into the breakfast area and there they were, my new friends from breakfast that morning. But now they had women with them. I walked over and they quickly invited me to join them. They were playing cards and drinking beer. I noticed a bottle of Jack Daniels along with lots of snack food on the table. I said let me go get some dry clothes on and I'll be right back down. I hurried up to my room, changed out of my wet clothes, and put on a Harley T-shirt and jeans, so I would fit in. I hurried back down to the lobby. What happened next can only be described as one of the funnest nights of my life. Rick and Debbie, Forrest and Sandra, John, Big Jim, Tina and Dale—we had so much fun! I don't know how we did not get thrown out of the hotel that night for excessive noise and having too much fun!

We even got the desk clerk involved. We asked her to come and take a group picture for us. She was a good sport and seemed more than willing to oblige. She took several pictures and returned to the front desk. When we looked at them, we all burst out laughing! She had the phone backwards and took pictures of herself! We called her back and she joined in the laughter with us when we showed her what she had done. She took some more pictures for us, this time with the camera pointed in the right direction.

They invited me to come to Virginia. Ride down and bring your husband they said. I said I would, but of course I knew I would probably never make a ride of that distance—or at least that's what I thought back in the summer of 2018.

We finally made our way to our separate rooms and crashed for the night. The next morning they must have gotten an early start, or slept in late, as I did not see them. I headed off to my meeting, on foot, just a few blocks away. At the conclusion of my meeting, I hustled out of Island Institute's office building and was going at a blistering pace down the crowded summer sidewalk toward the hotel. I had no time to spare as I had to be on the bike heading for home, 90 miles away, by 2pm. It was my only chance of catching the last ferry to Swan's Island that afternoon and I needed a little wiggle room to account for the busy summer traffic on Route 1. I hurried past the little shops, restaurants, and bars that dotted the main drag of Rockland. I was about a block away from the hotel when I heard, "DONNA!" I turned around and there was Big Jim standing outside a bar about half a block back. I doubled back and he gave me a big hug. He wanted me to come in and wanted to buy me a drink. He said the rest of the crew was inside. I told him I couldn't stay. I had less than 5 minutes to get on my bike and get underway or I would miss my ferry. He said, "Meeting you was the highlight of this trip." I was so touched. Another hug and I scurried off toward the hotel thinking I would never see Big Jim or the rest of the crew again.

As I made my way across the country, I was excited to reunite with my friends once I reached Virginia. When I arrived in Natural Bridge at the home of Rick and Debbie, it was a Sunday afternoon. They had the smoker going, a cooler full of beer, and they had invited everyone I met in Rockland,

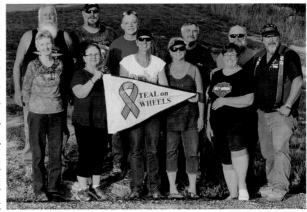

*Virginia Crew*

plus other friends and family to join us. Big Jim's wife, Vicki, was there. She had not been with the group in Maine and it was nice to meet her. Debbie prepared a wonderful spread of food for us to enjoy. The fun began from the moment I arrived. I stayed two nights with Rick and Debbie at their beautiful home. On Sunday night, after all of our eating and drinking, we all piled into the family van and went down the road to see the evening light show at the Natural Bridge. It is a great tourist attraction and is rich in history. It was formed when a cavern collapsed leaving a natural stone arch. It was surveyed by a young George Washington and owned by Thomas Jefferson in the 18th century. In 1927, President Calvin Coolidge inaugurated "The Drama of Creation," a light show that transformed the site into a night time destination. My first day and night with the Virginia Crew had been packed full of activity. I was happy to be in Natural Bridge with my friends.

On Monday, we went riding. They took me to the Blue Ridge Parkway and some other scenic places nearby. We stopped at the Peaks of Otter Lodge. The Peaks of Otter are three mountain peaks situated close together in the Blue Ridge Mountains overlooking the town of Bedford. It was great to be riding with my friends. The hospitality they showed me was so heartwarming. I may never see my Virginia crew again, but their love will be with me forever.

## *Chapter 20*

# TOO MANY DEATHS

**In early January 2021, I received an email** from Anne who runs the Turning the Tide Ovarian Cancer Retreat. Like so many other emails that I have received from Anne over the years, the subject read, *This is sad news.* Anne has the challenging job of notifying the women who attend the retreat when one of us has passed away. In the last two months, she has written to us four times to inform us of the deaths of Dawn, Kim, Alice, and now Becca. Becca was just 32 years old. She had a Master's Degree in Art Education. She was a young woman with a promising future until she was diagnosed with ovarian cancer. I met Becca at the 2019 Retreat. At that time, she was cautiously optimistic about her future. She had already been on a challenging journey with her cancer at that point. Becca died on January 2, 2021.

At times, I feel surrounded by death, my own impending

death, and that of others whom I don't think will survive. I think that I have become numb to it. I've accepted that death is a part of life, but it doesn't make the losses any easier. Death from cancer feels tragic—lives lost too soon.

As a part of the cancer community, I have many friends and acquaintances who are cancer patients. We are an unlikely band of sisters and brothers who are joined together by disease. We would not otherwise know one another, but our illness has brought us together. There's one bit of advice I often give to newly diagnosed cancer patients, I tell them to get a cancer buddy. Find someone with cancer, preferably the same type of cancer they have, someone who is further along in their journey, and use them as a resource. They are walking the walk, just like you. My husband Charlie has been amazing. My family and friends are great support, but they are not going through what I am going through. They have not experienced living with a terminal cancer diagnosis. There's so much that I don't share with them. I don't want to burden them with more worry. Charlie is a fixer. He likes to make things better, but he can't fix my cancer.

I have come to the conclusion that watching a loved one go through cancer is harder on family members and friends than it is for the patient. Because of that, I keep a lot to myself, and only share certain things with those who love me and care for me. I share the rest with my cancer buddies.

We receive the news of death now in many ways; phone calls, text messages, emails, social media posts, no matter how we find out, the moment we hear or read about a loss of life, we feel sadness. We pause and remember that person in our own way. I am writing this book during the time of Covid-19 and our country is sheltering in place from the pandemic. When someone dies now, during the time of Covid, we cannot gather to comfort one another and participate in normal end-of-life rituals. We must find our own ways to say goodbye.

My first experience with a cancer death was that of my maternal grandmother when I was in my early 20s. She was an amazingly lively lady and I think I take after her quite a bit. She worked as a secretary for a real estate company in Ocean City, NJ, at a law office in Norristown, PA, and for a steel company in Jeffersonville, PA. When the weekends came, she did fun stuff with us—all the time! She took us to museums in Philadelphia, to the zoo, and to the Jersey shore. We were always going some-where, always doing something fun. She also liked to drink beer and she smoked Camel non-filter cigarettes. I grew up in Skip-pack, PA, a small town about 35 miles northwest of Philadel-phia. My grandmother, who we called Gran, would come and pick me up along with her son, my uncle Don, who was only two years older than me and who lived with my family. When we weren't going off on some big adventure, she would take us with her to the local bar, the Dutch Cottage, located just minutes from my house. She would sit at the bar drinking her beer, and Don and I would sit at a nearby table eating little bags of potato chips and drinking cokes with cherries in the glass. Gran would give us change for the shuffleboard game and that would keep us busy for hours. I think I developed my love for beer because I wanted to be like my grandmother. She was not your typical grandmother of the 1960s—she dressed in hippie clothes. She wore bell bottom pants, wild print tunic tops, and always wore a dangling, oversized necklace of some sort. She didn't dress like that when she went to work, but on the weekends, she cut loose.

When Gran got sick and was diagnosed with lung cancer, (those damn Camel non-filter cigarettes), her death came quickly, in just a matter of a few weeks. She started treatment, but it was too late. She died in 1981 at the age of 68.

Treatments have improved over the years and many can-cer patients can survive for long periods with good quality of life. Some patients are cured, and some, like me, live with their can-cer like it's a chronic disease. We are programmed with a strong will to live, oftentimes foregoing quality of life to live longer. I don't think that will be me. I have often said, "I don't care how long I live, only how well I live." Quality of life is more important than length of life to me.

In the summer of 2017, I decided I was going to ride my

motorcycle, a maroon 2014 Harley Softail Deluxe, to visit all of the women from my ovarian cancer retreat who lived in Maine. I did not make it to see all of them, but I did get to visit many. It was great seeing them in their own homes and meeting some of their partners. I knew these women from the time I spent with them at the retreat, so seeing them in their home environment gave me more insight into their lives. My first visit was to Amherst to see Judith in her lovely log cabin home. Judith was my roommate at our first two retreats in 2016 and 2017. Next up was Diane who lived in an older home in Vassalboro. She was the "arts and crafts" lady at the retreat. She was lighthearted and fun. I traveled up north to Sherman to visit with Vicky. She was the person I most wanted to get to know when I arrived at my first retreat. She had a great laugh and a great command of the room when she was in it. She had a great passion for anything with a dragonfly on it. Dragonfly earrings, dragonfly T-shirt, even dragonfly socks! Next, I went south in the state to Scarborough, my first riding adventure on Route 95 and 295 through Portland. There I visited with Kathy in her beautiful home near Higgins Beach. All of these women had earned a place in my heart. They were my friends, my cancer buddies. They are all gone now—losing their lives to ovarian cancer, but not before bringing joy and love and laughter to this world.

Every year at the Turning the Tide Retreat, we gather down by the edge of Lake Damariscotta at Camp Kieve, in Nobleboro, Maine to remember and honor all of the previous retreat attendees who have lost their lives to cancer. Since the first year of the retreat, 2012, more than 50 women have died. Ovarian cancer ranks fifth in cancer deaths among women. The overall 5-year survival rate for all stages is 47%, meaning more than half of the women diagnosed with ovarian cancer will die in less than 5 years. I have stage IV ovarian cancer and the five-year survival rate is just 17%.

A few months ago, Dawn, one of my Turning the Tide sisters passed away. She was special, loved by everyone who met her. Dawn would make inspiring signs with encouraging words and decorate them with teal ribbons and bows. She made one sign that I was particularly fond of. It had an arrow pointing towards the person holding it. The sign said, ***This is what courage looks like.*** I picked it up and had my picture taken. It felt like I finally had a word that described all that I had been through, "COURAGE". Dawn had courage—incredible courage. On the day I met her at the retreat, she wanted to go kayaking on the lake. Everyone else who wanted to kayak had gone earlier in the day, including me. I told Dawn I'd go a second time. I couldn't think of anything more relaxing than paddling around the lake listening to the call of the distant loons. It was Dawn's first time kayaking. She caught on quickly. We chatted about all the different treatments she had tried. Dawn took a holistic approach in addition to traditional treatments. I had stayed on the traditional, pharmaceutical path. From the start, I admired Dawn's tenacity.

We reconnected after the retreat in May 2019 and shared a room with Margaret, another Turning the Tide sister, at the Stowe Weekend of Hope Cancer Conference in Vermont. Dawn, Margaret, and I stayed up until the wee hours of the morning sharing stories. One of the best stories Dawn shared was about a dead dog belonging to one of her co-workers. The guy enlisted Dawn's help when his dog died. He put the dog into a freezer when it died and went about making a casket for his beloved pet. When the casket was finally ready, the dog's owner removed the dog from the freezer. He was frozen stiff, not bendable in any way, and did not fit into the box. The dog had to be thawed out to get it into the casket. He kept calling Dawn each step of the way in a panic and Dawn would talk him through what he needed to do. The death of a human being, or a pet, is not funny business, but the way Dawn told the story was just so outrageous that Margaret and I laughed until we cried. Dawn was such a great storyteller. She got herself into situations like the dead dog scenario because she was too kind to ever say no.

As Dawn neared the end of her life, she was an inpatient at a hospital in Boston. She was being transferred to a stand-alone hospice facility. She was stopping all curative treatment. Dawn and Anne Tonachel had grown very close over the years, so Anne would be riding with Dawn in the ambulance and Dawn's husband would be waiting for their arrival at the hospice facility. Anne sent an email after Dawn got settled into her room with a picture of Dawn. I didn't want to open it. I didn't want my last memory of Dawn to be looking frail. I wanted to remember her on the lake at the retreat, or at Stowe telling funny stories. I finally opened the email and the attached picture popped up. It was Dawn in her bed with a clear glass bowl on her lap. It was filled with scoops and scoops of chocolate ice cream—more than any big-sized man could eat, let alone a woman in the final days of her life. Anne shared that Dawn, always one to make the best of any situation, had declared, "This place is great! They have 24/7 chocolate ice cream!" Dawn died four days later.

The day after Dawn's death in early November, 2020, I got on my motorcycle, hopped on the ferry, and went to the mainland. I stopped in Ellsworth at a floral shop to buy some

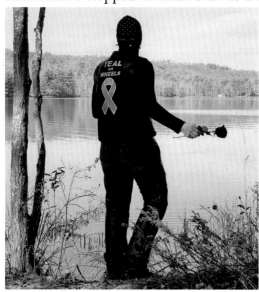

*Throwing roses for Dawn at Lake Damariscotta*

long stem red roses. I asked the clerk to cut the stems shorter so I could fit them in my motorcycle's saddlebag. I rode 110 miles to Camp Kieve where our Retreat is held each year. This was the place where I had met Dawn when we went kayaking together on the lake. It only seemed appropriate that this was where I should say goodbye to Dawn. I parked my motorcycle just above the Kennedy Learning Center, the main lodge. Just down the hillside was the fire pit, next to the lake where we held our memorial service each year. As I made my way down, holding tightly to the roses, I expected to see all the other women, but I was alone. I had never been to the camp without my Turning the Tide sisters. A few of the chairs by the fire pit were overturned. I set all the chairs upright and evenly spaced them out around the pit. I knew no one else would be joining me that day, but in my mind and in my heart, they were all there with me. It was warm for a November day in Maine and the lake was like glass on the surface. I sat for a spell and shared some thoughts out loud about Dawn. Then I approached the lake and threw the six roses, one by one into the lake. I watched in silence as they sat on the surface of the water, barely moving away from the shoreline. Goodbye, my friend.

I've lost other friends to other types of cancer. My motorcycle friend Howard lost his life to liver cancer shortly after being diagnosed. Diana fought against metastatic breast cancer for many years before losing her battle. Rusty, who took me lobstering with him for two seasons, died of lung cancer after just a few months. Erich, who was diagnosed with liver, pancreatic, and colon cancer, continued on in his professional music career until he no longer could, in the end donating his body to science. Sue, who traveled across the country from Maine to California searching for a cure, died from pancreatic cancer. Sharon, my childhood friend, invited me to share her last vacation in the Florida Keys with her and her family less than two weeks before her death from lung cancer. My neighbors from Swan's Island, Christie, age 32, just starting out her married life, and Bud, age 60, a hard working islander, passed within months of one another from colon cancer. My friend Paula, who lived the healthiest of lifestyles, died of liver cancer just a few short months after being diagnosed. There are others, way too many others, whose lives have impacted me.

When I lose a friend to cancer, or any form of death, I try not to get stuck in my grief. I've had that happen at times over the years and it is a hard place to be. I'm able to give myself permission to pause and acknowledge the death, to remember our friendship, to say goodbye, and then move on. I tell myself that the person I lost would not want me to continue in my sadness, but that they would want me to go on living a joyous life in their absence. I choose joy and happiness as my way of honoring and celebrating them and I want my family and friends to do the same when I am gone.

*Chapter 21*

# OLD FRIENDS

**About 5 months before I left** on my Teal on Wheels trip I was back home in Pennsylvania for my niece Cera's wedding. I do not come from a particularly close knit family, so events like weddings and funerals are occasions where I get to see other family members. Cera's wedding was not your typical church affair, but rather a casual, outdoor event. At the end of the day, the bride and groom were happily married and I got to reconnect with some of my family members. I'm sure the celebration continued well after dark, but Charlie and I politely said our goodbyes and headed to our next social obligation—a pizza and beer party at the home of our friends, Larry and Denise. Larry and I go all the way back to kindergarten. We share a special bond of sorts, Larry's last name is Emel and my maiden name was Emmell, both pronounced the same way. For more than five decades, we have bantered back and forth about which spelling was correct. The misspelling of Larry's last name, and the correct spelling of mine, has forever bonded us together. Denise joined us when we entered junior high, after having attended Catholic elementary school. Larry and Denise were not high school sweethearts, but connected at one of our high school reunions, and the rest, as they say, is history—married with three sons, who all spell their last name wrong, too. Over the years, we had lost touch, but a few years back Larry contacted me to tell me that they had rented a house on Swan's Island with their friends, Carol and Brian, and they would be vacationing on my island for a week. Our friendship was renewed and a new friendship began when I met Carol and Brian that summer.

When we arrived at Larry and Denise's house after the wedding, a whole gang of old friends, along with Carol and Brian, were present. My old school friends, Jennie, Wendy, and Donna (Denise's twin sister) were there with their husbands, Mike, Jim, and Chris. I had a special relationship with each of the women. Jennie was, and is, my oldest friend. We have known each other for more than 55 years. Our fathers were both truck drivers and they were friends, so Jennie and I became friends before we even started school. Wendy was my best friend in high school. We were co-captains of the Perkiomen Valley High School varsity girls' basketball team. Wendy was the better athlete. We were good friends, both on and off the court. Our friendship started in the 7th grade when we arrived at junior high school from two different elementary schools. We knew of each other from playing basketball against one another during our elementary school days. We were both very competitive and it was an honor to be co-captain with Wendy when we became seniors. I didn't know Donna, Denise's sister, all that well in school, but our paths crossed after college when we worked together as laboratory technologists at the same hospital in Pennsylvania. We also played recreational volleyball together in our 20s and 30s.

Seated in Larry and Denise's living room, eating pizza and drinking beer, I shared with my old friends my idea of Teal on Wheels. I felt like they thought my idea was fantastic. They greeted it with enthusiasm and all promised to support my cause. After all, they were my friends and that's what friends do—support one another.

A few months went by and my Teal on Wheels plans were being solidified. I had the bike. I was working on my message of raising awareness about ovarian cancer. And, I was in the midst of fundraising. A strange thing happened—as people started to support my cause with financial donations—only Carol and Brian, the newest of my friends, made a donation. But what about Larry and Denise, Jennie and Mike, Wendy and Jim, Donna and Chris? I felt let down by the inaction of my friends—friends that I thought I could count on. My feelings were hurt. I knew these friends as generous, kind, and caring, but I guess they had forgotten their promise to me.

One night my phone rang and it was Jennie. I could hear chatter and laughter in the background and that seemed odd. I wondered where she was calling from.

She said, "Guess who's here with me?" I had no idea. She started naming off everybody; Larry, Denise, Wendy, Donna…. everybody was there together. I thought why are they calling me. Jennie asked me where I would be, along my way on my trip across the country on Sunday, September 29. I replied, "I hope I'll be home by then." She said, "We need you to be in Royersford, Pennsylvania that day." I said, "What?"

Jennie went on to explain that my friends, my generous, kind, caring friends were putting together a beef and beer fundraiser for me, to support Teal on Wheels. She went on to say that they wanted me to join them that day to celebrate my ride. The group had reached out to other high school friends to ask them to support the event—to sponsor a keg of beer or food, or just make a monetary donation. They had a DJ—Joe, from our high school class, who volunteered to DJ the event. It sounded amazing! Here they were, all my friends, working hard to help me reach my $50,000 fundraising goal and I thought they had forgotten all about me. How could I have doubted them? I confessed. I told them, "I thought you were all a bunch of cheapskates when you didn't send me any money!" They all laughed.

It would take some adjusting in my ride schedule, but I assured them that I could be in Pennsylvania on September 29 and it would be my honor to join them that day.

As my trip across the country progressed, I realized I was way ahead of schedule and arrived in Pennsylvania on the Tuesday before the big event. I stayed in Gettysburg on Tuesday night and traveled only as far as York the following day where I toured the Harley-Davidson manufacturing plant. It was awesome seeing all the beautiful motorcycles being assembled and painted and finally shipped out the door of the plant to Harley dealerships across the country. What I wouldn't give for a brand new, shiny, no scratches, beast of a machine with all the bells and whistles! I doubted that I would ever pull the trigger on a brand new bike again, but it was fun to dream about it.

I left the Harley-Davidson plant in the pouring rain and headed east on Route 30. A nice 18-wheel truck driver followed me down the highway offering protection from the speeding traffic behind me. When it's raining hard, I ride slower. My vision is seriously impaired. There are no windshield wipers on a bike or on your helmet making riding in the rain challenging. I used to ride super slow in the rain, but years of experience have now given me confidence in my bike's traction and my own ability to handle my bike on wet roads.

I decided I didn't really want to ride in the rain any longer. I had plenty of time to make it to the east side of the state before Sunday, so I got off Route 30, near Lancaster, and got a room in Montvale. Spending the night in Montvale would give me an opportunity to get some laundry done and arrive in Royersford the next day with a full compliment of clean clothes. It would be my last time doing laundry on the road before arriving home in Maine.

When I arrived in Royersford the next day, my first stop was WAWA, a chain mini-mart store and gas station. There are no WAWA convenience stores in Maine and I wanted a sandwich on one of those fresh WAWA rolls. I got some lunch and went out to the back of the parking lot where I had parked my bike. I sat on a curb to eat my tasty meal. When I finished I got to work deciding where I would stay. I decided to get a hotel room for three nights since I would not be leaving the area until Monday morning. I splurged and got a room at a nice hotel just outside of town in Linfield. This would be convenient to all of the visiting I was planning to do while I was in the area. Charlie would be arriving the next day—riding down to Pennsylvania from Maine to join me for the fundraiser and to accompany me the last 600 miles back home. I was looking forward to seeing him when he arrived on Saturday, September 28. I had last seen him on September 9 when we parted ways in Moab, Utah, thousands of miles ago. He had headed back to Salt Lake City to fly home and I had headed east toward Colorado.

Charlie had been suffering with a bad head cold for a few days before leaving Maine and I was nervous about sharing a room with him for three nights. The last thing I needed was to get sick on the final leg of my journey. I was also worried about him riding all the way to Pennsylvania when he was not feeling 100%. But he arrived on Saturday as expected and it was great to see him again.

We had planned to ride our motorcycles to the fundraising event on Sunday, which was being held at the VFW on South 4th Avenue in Royersford. We would stay for a little while, so everyone could see my teal and white Harley, then have someone follow us back to the ho-

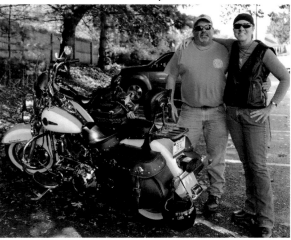

*Charlie and me arriving at the fundraiser*

tel, where we would leave the bikes and return with a designated driver, so we could enjoy the festivities of the day without worrying about drinking and riding the bikes. Our friend Scott volunteered to be our driver. Scott and his wife Jen were good friends from our younger days. Whenever we returned to Pennsylvania, no matter the reason, we always visited with them.

The event was wonderful—so many supporters turned out to greet me! There were old high school friends from more than 40 years earlier, college friends, former co-workers, three of the four people that were in our wedding, our old volleyball gang, Charlie's family and my family—it was so good to see everybody.

There was music and food, and lots of beer. I may have concentrated too much on the beer and too little on the food. I realized that much too late in the day and thought for sure it would impact the next day's riding, but surprisingly it did not. I was thoroughly enjoying myself reuniting with old friends and sharing stories of my time on the road. At one point, a déjà vu experience occurred. The DJ had everybody gather in a circle, maybe it was for the "chicken dance", but the next thing I knew I was up on top of a picnic table dancing and inviting my best friend Jennie's granddaughter, McKenzie, up on the table with me to dance. McKenzie is the cutest little girl. She was very shy about climbing up there with me, but her mom encouraged her and up she came. Before long Charlie jumped up on the table and McKenzie got down. This is the déjà vu part—at our wedding, Charlie and I climbed up onto a table and were dancing. These two table dances were 28 years apart. If the frequency in opportunities to table dance only occur every 28 years, I doubt that I will ever enjoy dancing on a table again in my lifetime.

At one point, my friend Jennie, who appeared to be the hostess of the event, was given the microphone from the DJ to say a few words. She invited me to come up front with her. We have been friends for over 55 years and although we took different paths in life, we have never lost touch with each other. Jennie is my longest, dearest friend. We know stuff about each other that we would probably never share with any of our other friends.

Everybody needs someone like that in their lives.

Jennie has been involved with the American Cancer Society's annual Relay for Life for more than 30 years. She knows how to raise money—who to ask, how to ask, and how to get it done. Jennie lost her youngest sister, Sharon, to lung cancer in 2017 at the age of 53. She also helped me get through my first cancer journey, cervical cancer in 1990. Here she was continuing her good work by helping me get closer to my fundraising goal.

With mic in hand, Jennie honored me by sharing some stories from our past. She had a few note cards to help her stay on point. When Jennie was done speaking, I took the mic and thanked everyone for working so hard to make this day so special for me. Raising money was just one part of the day, but getting to see so many people from so many different parts of my life was the biggest reward of the day. My friends had raised almost $6,000 to help me get closer to my fundraising goal. I couldn't believe it—just a few months earlier I was thinking they had all forgotten me. I was so wrong. I was sad that the day had to come to an end. It was hard to say goodbye to everyone that had come out to cheer me on. I didn't know if I would ever see some of them again, but I was glad I got to see them on that day, at that event. My heart was filled with love—what a wonderful life I have lived!

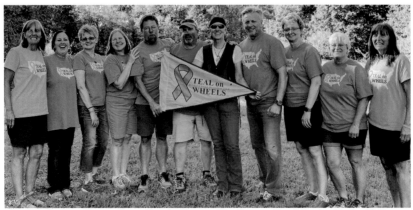

*Denise, Donna, Donna Jane, Jennie, Larry, Charlie, me, Joe, Wendy, Cindy & Donna*
*(Donna was a popular name back in the 1960s when I was born)*

# *Chapter 22*

# KINDNESS MATTERS

**Teal on Wheels started out as my idea,** but it would not have been possible without an army of people supporting me. I would never have completed the journey, or even started it, without the help of so many. Their enthusiasm and their energy—that's what kept me moving forward and allowed me to turn my idea into reality.

I want you to meet some of my supporters. Some helped in small ways, others in bigger ways, but I needed everyone, working together, to get me from the starting line to the finish.

Once I finally had my teal and white Harley in my possession, I needed an inspection and a thorough mechanical evaluation along with routine maintenance before I ventured out on my journey across the country. My mechanic, Stanley Gardner, owner of Gardner Racing Concepts (GRC), located just outside of Ellsworth, was the man I needed to see. Stanley takes stock motorcycles and makes them go fast. He builds motors for racing bikes and is a motorcycle drag racer himself. I didn't need to go fast, I just needed my bike to be reliable. The last thing I wanted was to break down on the road somewhere in the middle of nowhere. Stanley had always treated me well whenever I took my Softail Deluxe in for servicing, so I called him up and told him what I was planning to do with my new bike. I explained that I wanted to be sure the bike was in perfect working order for the trip. I made an appointment and took the bike in for servicing. At GRC, you can go into the garage and watch the work being done on your bike. I like that. It gives you a better idea of what goes on behind the scenes in a garage, and sometimes you learn

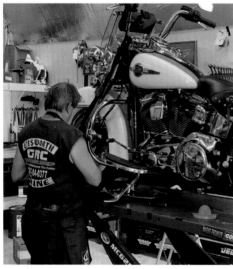

things about your motorcycle. I watched while Stanley and his employee, Erik, were hard at work, changing my spark plug, adjusting air pressure, installing a new air filter, checking brakes and lights, giving the bike a thorough going over. At one point, Stanley approached where I was sitting and watching. He had two small boxes in his hands. He looked me straight in the eye and said,

*Stanley working on my motorcycle*

"You seem like somebody who cares about the environment." I replied, "I do, Stanley." I didn't know where he was headed with his statement. He went on to show me the two different types of oil filters he had in the boxes, explaining one was a throw away type, you get a new filter each time you get an oil change. The other, the one that was much better for the environment, was a reusable oil filter. It would need to be cleaned with each oil change, but the filter itself would be reused over and over. I do care about the environment, so I chose the reusable oil filter. Even if I didn't care about it, I would have been afraid not to choose the reusable oil filter—I didn't want to disappoint Stanley. When Stanley was done with servicing my bike, he lowered the jack and rolled the bike out of the shop. I followed him to the office and asked him how much I owed him. He said, "Nothing." I said, "What?" He replied, "No charge, I want to help you with your trip." I told him that I thought that was extremely generous, but that I wasn't comfortable riding away without paying. I countered with, "Can I at least pay for the parts you used?" Stanley said, "No." I don't know how much the parts and service that day were worth, hundreds and hundreds of dollars, I'm sure. I was so grateful for the kindness that Stanley showed me—forever solidifying my loyalty as a lifelong customer and taking our relationship to a new level, adding friendship to our already existing mechanic-customer relationship.

I could not get an inspection at GRC, Stanley doesn't inspect bikes, so I went to see Les Foss, a friend of Stanley's who owns Island Towing and Auto Repair in Town Hill. Les was a biker dude that liked to go fast. I had met Les many years earlier at my favorite barbeque joint, Mainely Meat, located about a quarter mile from his garage. I would often stop there in the summer for takeout and Les would be sitting at the bar having lunch. We talked bikes while I was waiting for my order to be ready. I pulled into the parking lot at Les' garage and went into the office. Les was seated behind the counter. As I approached I started telling him about my trip and my new bike. Les knew all about it. He told me he had already contributed a bunch of money to my trip. He went on to explain that every Friday at Mainely Meat they were giving away their "Max Platter"—a huge tray of ribs, pulled pork, smoked chicken and all the sides. He told me they had a big jar with TEAL on WHEELS written on the side. If you made a donation, you got to put your name on a slip of paper and into the jar it went. This got you a chance to win the weekly feast. Les told me that over the last few weeks he had put lots of money in the jar, but had not yet won a Max Platter. I was un-

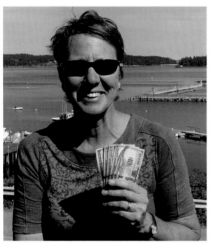
*$500 donated by Mainely Meat BBQ*

aware of this fundraising event going on at Mainely Meat, but was touched by what they were doing for me. A few weeks later, Charlie stopped at Mainely Meat for take-out. Maxine, our favorite waitress, gave him an envelope with a $500 donation towards Teal on Wheels. I was amazed by who was supporting me and the creative ways by which they were doing it.

Back to the inspection, Les came out from behind the counter and out to my bike. He looked it over. Everything was in good working order and he wrote out the inspection paperwork and applied the inspection sticker to my bike's plate. I asked him how much I owed him, and just like Stanley, he said, "Nothing." Another random act of kindness. Again, I was grateful to know such wonderful people.

Financial donations starting at $5, and capping in the thousands, came from an amazingly generous group of supporters. Many donations came through the GoFundMe platform. Other donations were sent directly to the Beth C. Wright Cancer Resource Center designated for Teal on Wheels. A few folks got creative with their fundraising efforts, like Mainely Meat and my old high school friends who had hosted a beef and beer fundraiser style event. My friend Deb, who lived on Swan's Island, started making teal turk's head bracelets, a traditional sailor's knot bracelet made of a variable number of interwoven strands of string. Deb made a big sign with a picture of me and my bike, and each week she would set up her little display at the island's craft fair in front of the old Methodist Church. Deb had a suggested donation of $10 for a bracelet. The bracelets took off like crazy and she found herself working day and night to keep up with demand. In the end, Deb donated over $1,000 to Teal on

Wheels. That was a lot of turk's head bracelets!

My community of Swan's Island has always been very generous when someone is sick or a personal tragedy has befallen someone. When I was first diagnosed with ovarian cancer, in the spring of 2016, several women stepped up and hosted a

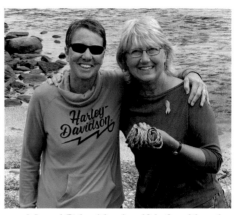

*Me and Deb with a handful of teal bracelets*

potluck benefit supper at the Odd Fellows Hall on the island. Typically, the person whom the benefit is being held for does not attend the supper. I would imagine it would feel uncomfortable being there watching people put money in the jar, box, or basket, whatever the collection vessel is at the entryway. Like others before me, I did not attend my benefit supper. When the basket of money, cash and checks, was delivered to my house by Jil, I was completely overwhelmed. Personal notes, cards, checks and cash filled the basket. I am not an overly emotional person. I have only cried twice since my cancer journey began, once at Dana Farber in Boston. The second time was the day I returned home from attending my first Turning the Tide Ovarian Cancer Retreat. I didn't just cry that day, I had a complete nuclear meltdown—everything that I had been keeping inside for the months came flooding out like a tsunami. The day that Jil dropped off the basket and a framed "Get Well" message signed by everyone who attended the supper, I cried for a third time. My tears that day as I went through the outpouring of love and money contained in the basket were tears of joy. I was grateful to live in such a giving community.

My friends Chris and Mary also came to my aid early on in my cancer journey. They started a GoFundMe page, where friends and family from near and far, generously opened their hearts and their wallets to support Charlie and me. I was filled with gratitude for the many people who supported us.

In preparing for Teal on Wheels, I saw a similar outpouring from my neighbors. Jil, once again, rose to the challenge, and secretly prepared a send off at the ferry terminal on the day I was leaving the island to begin my trip. She asked everyone to assemble at the ferry terminal and to wear something teal. Flags and signs were encouraged. Jil prepared a large banner that required three people to hold it up. Of course, it was teal and read, GO DONNA in huge letters. In smaller letters, it read, Teal on

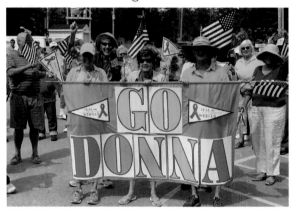

*Departing Swan's Island for the start of my trip*

Wheels Ovarian Cancer Awareness Tour with teal ribbons. As we pulled down the road toward our spot in the ferry waiting line, I could see the animated crowd awaiting my arrival. This was fantastic! I got out of the car and greeted my wellwishers. I was so pleased to receive this unexpected send off. Hugs, cheers, and good luck wishes continued as I worked my way through the crowd trying to acknowledge everyone who was there. It was great to see so many smiling faces, my friends and neighbors saying goodbye and good luck. I would not see them again for more than a month.

I had one island family in particular, consisting of several generations, that became some of my biggest supporters. I received a cash donation from Les and his wife, Rhonda, one day in the ferry line. Les' sisters, Jean and Norene, and his brother, Tim, each made a donation. Les and Rhonda's daughters, Lesley and Leah, showed up at my house one day. The sisters, both in their 20s, make their living on the ocean lobstering. Leah had a very generous check made out to me and her older sister Lesley sat at my kitchen table and endorsed one of her lobstering paychecks, making it payable to me. I was overwhelmed by these two young women showing their support for my cause. This whole family amazed me. When I arrived home from my trip, after 40 days on the road, I was a couple thousand dollars shy of my $50,000 fundraising goal. I made a last ditch plea on my Facebook page to see if I could get to the $50,000 goal. People responded, some giving a second time. I updated my Facebook page as each new donation came in. When I was just $447 shy of my goal, Jean's car pulled in my driveway and she came to my back door. I opened the door to greet her. She handed me $447 in cash and announced, "Here's what you need to make your $50,000 goal." We do not have a bank on Swan's Island or an ATM, so I wondered where Jean could have gotten the money. She told me she went to see her brother Les, who at the time was a lobster dealer on the island. She told him she needed $447 for me and he gave Jean the money, or gave it to me, really.

When I first started raising money, I realized I needed a way to manage it. I did not want to be responsible for it and felt the need for complete transparency. There was a brief time early on when the idea of creating a 501c3 non-profit for Teal on Wheels was on the table. The effort would require a lot of work, but mostly it required time, something I had very little of. From the start of the project: securing the bike, fundraising, and planning the trip, shipping my motorcycle, leaving the island to fly to the West Coast, getting on the motorcycle and starting to ride—everything had to happen quickly. I had a little over three months to get it all done and establishing a new non-profit for a one time event just didn't make sense.

Managing all of the donations that came in for Teal on Wheels was a big job, which fell onto Michael Reisman at the Beth C. Wright Cancer Resource Center. It was critical for the success and transparency that I had someone like Michael helping me. I set up the GoFundMe online account to automatically transfer donations directly to the Beth C. Wright Cancer Resource Center's bank account every two weeks. Checks and cash that I received would also go to Michael to manage. I felt like a drug dealer dropping off envelopes full of cash and checks to whomever was behind the desk when I showed up at the Ellsworth Center. Some checks were made out to me personally, so I had to cash them first and put the money into my zippered blue bank bag until I could make the drop off.

About a month after the trip was over, I met with Michael and we went over all the finances. In the end, I had selected several ovarian cancer non-profit organizations to receive donations as a result of my efforts. First and foremost, and nearest and dearest to my heart, was Turning the Tide Ovarian Cancer Retreat. I presented Anne Tonachel, the director, with one of the big cardboard checks at the 2019 Retreat, held in November, a month after the completion of my trip. I also donated to Ovations for the Cure, National Ovarian Cancer Coalition, and Ovarian Cancer Research Alliance. In the end, enough money had been raised to make a donation to the Beth C. Wright Cancer Resource Center for all that they had done to help me financially manage Teal on Wheels. Without the help of Michael Reisman and the Center, I could not have done what I did.

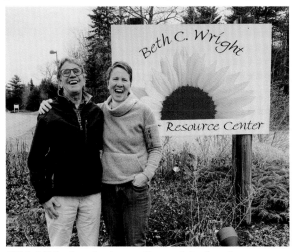

*With Michael on the day we dispersed the donations*

There are simply too many people to thank for their part, big or small, in making Teal on Wheels a success. Each and every person who had a hand in supporting me and my efforts deserves to be acknowledged—from those who supported my fundraising efforts to the kind and caring people I met during my cross country travels—some generously paid for my meal after hearing my story. One of the best meals I had on my trip was at the Black

Bison Pub in Syracuse, Kansas. I had had a tough day of riding up across the Monarch Pass, 11,312 feet in elevation, to cross the Rocky Mountains and into Kansas. The wind was unbelievable that day and I was glad to be off the bike and enjoying a delicious steak dinner. The owner of the pub was a breast cancer survivor and after hearing my story, she reached across the bar where I was sitting and picked up the credit card slip when the barmaid placed it in front of me. She crumbled it up and said, "Your meal is on the house." I was met with this type of kindness all across the country.

*Chapter 23*

# GOING HOME

**When I reached Pennsylvania** on my Teal on Wheels ride, I had a lot of extra time waiting for the beef and beer fundraiser my friends were hosting. That gave me a chance to spend some time reliving some of my childhood and teen years by visiting my hometown of Skippack. I pulled my motorcycle to the side of the road in front of my childhood home, a red brick, two-story house, with an attached garage. It looked different, smaller than I remembered it. But one thing remained the same, the two big sycamore trees in front that I spent hours climbing as a young girl. One of the fun things about the sycamore trees was the bark. It looked like camouflage and was easy to peel off in large strips. I spent endless hours up in those two trees as a child. I also stopped at the small church in the center of the town to visit the gravesite of my friend, Richie, who tragically lost his life in a car crash my senior year of high school. I rode past the Dutch Cottage, the bar where my grandmother took me when I was a little girl. It's now known at The Dutch Tavern. The main street of my childhood town was lined with little shops and eateries. Many things looked familiar, but just as many had changed.

The time I got to spend in Pennsylvania on my trip brought back a lot of memories for me. It was a going home moment. It was hard to leave, but I had a new home in Maine, and I needed to get back to my life there. I didn't know if I would ever get back to Pennsylvania again, but I would hold the many smiling faces, conversations, hugs, and kisses from friends and family dearly in my memory. My heart was full as Charlie and I got ready to hit the road.

We would have a long day of riding north. We were heading to New York and decided the best route to get there would be to take the Pennsylvania Turnpike. We could hop on at the Lansdale exit of the Northeast extension of the turnpike and head straight north. The sky was overcast and we were hoping not to encounter any rain. We made our way to the turnpike entrance, the first toll road of my entire trip. We began to ride north. Immediately we noticed all the construction and concrete barriers on the edge of the inside lane. It started to rain, but there was no safe place to pull over and don our rain gear. We continued on. I was in the lead and looking for anyplace to pull off and gear up, but the construction barriers prevented us from pulling off to the side of the road. The rain was cold and I didn't want to ride hundreds of miles in wet clothing. Finally, we stopped on the side of the road under an overpass as cars and trucks went zooming by. We donned our rain gear and continued on our way.

We traveled north into New York and by that time the rain was coming down in buckets. I could hardly see a thing ahead of me. My glasses had fogged up, and we were getting hammered by rain. It was not safe to continue riding in these conditions. I got off at the next exit. At the stop sign, I could see a small convenience store and gas station directly across the intersection. I pulled into the parking lot and parked right next to the building. I got off the bike and huddled up against the building under an overhang. I just wanted to get out of the rain for a few minutes. Charlie followed my lead. We stood there in our helmets, thankful to be off our motorcycles and safe. We consulted our map. We had originally been planning to meet up with our friends, Jim and Carrie, at their home in the Adirondacks. Rain was in the forecast for the next few days, so we scrapped the idea of going to the Adirondacks and had to come up with a plan B. We decided to head to Schenectady instead. It seemed like the rain was letting up a little, so we got back on our bikes and made our way back to Interstate 88 East. After 229 miles, we called it quits, 67 miles short of Schenectady. We had ridden about 200 miles in the rain that day and just wanted to be done and off the bikes. We ended up in Oneonta for the night. We got into our hotel room, warmed up, and ordered pizza delivery so we didn't have to go back out in the rain again.

We left Oneonta the next morning in a light rain and made our way to White River Junction, VT. The further north we rode, the colder it was getting and the rain didn't help. I was chilled by the time we finished our day of riding. The long trip had taken a lot out of me. I was tired of riding in the rain and tired of being cold. We decided to stay in White River for two nights and wait out the rain. I longed for one of the dry, hot days of riding in southern Utah.

While staying in White River Junction, I got a call on my cell phone from a Maine reporter from the Bangor Daily News. The reporter, Nick Sambides, was writing a story about my Teal on Wheels cross country trip. My plan to raise awareness about ovarian cancer was working. The more press I got, the more information about this deadly cancer was getting out there. I was pleased to chat with Nick who told me the story would run in the Bangor Daily News on October 4, a couple days later.

We left White River Junction on October 3. It was 42 degrees when we started riding that morning and topped out at 53 degrees that afternoon. Charlie wanted to find the Cornish-Windsor Bridge that spanned the Connecticut River between Windsor,

201

VT and Cornish, NH. He promised that it would not be too far out of our way. The bridge was built in 1866 and is the longest two-span covered bridge in the world according to the sign there. The 460-foot structure was built using a lattice truss system. It was originally a toll bridge, but in 1943 it was made toll-free by the state of New Hampshire. As we approached the bridge, I was excited to ride through it, but once inside, my excitement turned to fear. The riding surface of the bridge was large timbers, with sharp edges sticking up. The surface was very uneven. It was extremely uncomfortable under the tires of my motorcycle. When we got to the far side and into New Hampshire, we stopped at a parking area to take some pictures. I was glad to be safely through the bridge. Charlie informed me that we had to go back through it to continue on our trip north. We had only ridden through just to say we did it and now had to turn around and go back through it again. I put up some resistance and said we

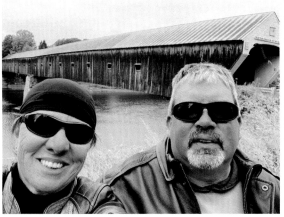

*Charlie and me at the Cornish-Windsor Bridge*

could just find a different route to Maine. In the end, Charlie won and we rode back through the bridge. I did not enjoy it one bit.

As we continued to make our way northeast, our ride took us to one of the most visited locations in New Hampshire during the fall foliage season—the Kancamagus Scenic Byway, simply known as "The Kanc". It is a 34.5 mile scenic drive along NH Route 112 in northern New Hampshire. It is well known as one of the best fall foliage viewing areas in the country and to our good fortune, it was October 3, nearly peak fall foliage season in New England. The Kanc cuts through the White Mountains National Forest. The views were spectacular—the reds, oranges, and yellows of the foliage against the deep green of the forest were breathtaking.

We left the Kanc behind and headed towards Conway, NH and the Maine border. We crossed into Maine at Fryeburg, happy to be

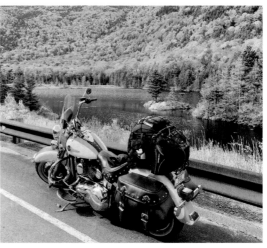

*Along the Kancamagus Scenic Byway*

back in our home state. As the trip was drawing to a close, I felt both sadness and happiness. Sadness to be nearing the end of the biggest adventure of my life, but happy to be getting home and going back to my normal life.

We headed to Augusta, our state's capital, for the night. As we came through Auburn on our way to Lewiston for a stop at the L-A Harley dealer, we were sitting at a traffic light. I had my Teal on Wheels vest on over my leather jacket. A small blue car pulled up alongside of me honking the horn. The passenger side window went down. The woman driver was hollering out her passenger side window at me. I had my ear buds in listening to my tunes and couldn't make out what she was saying. I turned my music off and she was still shouting. She was telling me that she had followed my trip across the country on Facebook. I thought to myself, WOW, I'm famous! She sent me a message on Facebook later that night. Her name was Sally and she rides a Harley trike.

We made it to Augusta. We were so close to home, but we would have to wait a little longer. Charlie had made arrangements for some of our riding friends to meet us to ride the last leg of the trip home. The group were my old friends from the Widows Sons Motorcycle Riding Association—the guys who had been with me at the start of the Teal on Wheels fundraising. I couldn't wait to see them again and ride home with them. They couldn't meet up with us until Saturday, so our arrival home would be delayed by a day. We spent Friday visiting the Maine State Museum in Augusta, four floors of the history of Maine. It was fascinating. When we finished up the Museum tour, we went to the car wash and washed our bikes. We wanted them to look good for the next day—our last day of the ride. We would be riding with our friends from Augusta to Ellsworth to the Lygonia Lodge. Reporters from WABI-TV5 in Bangor and the Mount Desert Islander newspaper would be waiting for our arrival. Great, more press coverage equaled raising more awareness for my cause.

After washing the bikes, we stopped into a convenience store for some drinks and snacks. As I was standing in line waiting to pay, Charlie noticed the newspaper stand, which had that day's edition of the Bangor Daily News. I was on the front page of the paper—a picture of me and my bike from southern Utah and a headline stating, 'I have completed something that was bigger than me'—a quote from my interview. I grabbed the newspaper and saw a second, larger picture on the bottom of the front page. It was me, standing at the edge of the lake at Crater Lake National Park in Oregon showing the back of my Teal on Wheels vest with the large teal cancer ribbon. WOW, I was the front page featured story! The article continued from the front page to section B3, where a third picture accompanied the rest of the story. I could not contain

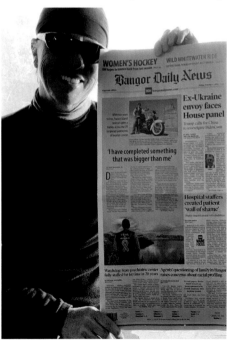

*Made the front page of the Bangor Daily News*

my excitement and turned to the people waiting in line to pay, announcing, "Hey, this is me. I made the front page of the paper." No one seemed all that impressed, but I surely was.

I awoke early the next morning and began to get ready for my final day of riding. I looked out the hotel window and saw frost on the roof. I wondered how cold it was outside. I started lugging my gear down to the bike and found the seats of our motorcycles covered in a hard frost. They were parked in the shade and it would be a while before the sun reached them. I scraped the frost off my seat. It was 38 degrees—another day of cold riding. We weren't meeting the Widows Sons riders until 10am in the parking lot of a nearby lumber company just east of Augusta. Hopefully, it would warm up some by then. We only had about a 10 minute ride to get to the meeting place. Some of the riders coming to meet us were leaving from Downeast Maine and would be riding for hours before getting to the rendezvous point. They would be cold. We arrived first and were waiting when we saw a group of motorcycles approaching from the east. We could hear the familiar rumble of their Harley engines. They pulled in and it was so good to see this band of brothers and sisters there to greet me and take me home. Mike, who I had bought the teal and white Harley from just a few months earlier, arrived in a convertible with the top down. He claimed his motorcycle wouldn't start that morning, but we all poked fun at him saying it was probably just too cold for him to ride. Scott and his wife, Veronica, had probably ridden the farthest. They told me they left home at 6am in the dark and it was only 30 degrees when they started their ride. One of the Widows Sons, my friend Howard, was dressed in a pair of insulated overalls. He reminded me of Randy from the Christmas Story movie—all bundled up and hardly able to move. My friend Joe, a big bear of a man from Downeast Maine was there. Joe was the man that gave me the $200 for my ride on the first day he ever met me. James, Adam, and Scott were also there. Others had similar stories of early starts and riding in the cold to get to the meeting place in time. Our friends, Aaron and Erica, were the last to arrive. Erica looked like she was half frozen. Her husband, Aaron, had told her it wouldn't be all that cold, so she hadn't put on any long underwear under her jeans or any leather chaps over them. What a great group of people— why would these people do this for me I wondered. I was hoping the day would continue to warm up and that we would have a great ride to Ellsworth.

I hugged them all and thanked them for coming to ride with me. They commented that it was an honor to escort me home—I felt that it was an honor to be riding in their company. Scott was selected to lead the ride and the plan was that I would ride second. He would let me take the lead when we approached the Lygonia Lodge and I would lead the way in. Scott set a comfortable pace for the one hundred miles we would be traveling together. Mike, in his convertible, followed our pack of ten bikes, protecting us from the rear. So much of my riding is solo, but there's something exhilarating about riding as part of a group of motorcycles. Riding with those riders, on that day, felt like the best thing ever.

As we were approaching the Lodge, a location I had only been to once before and on that occasion I had come from the opposite direction, Scott slowed down and motioned me to take the lead. We were almost there. Would there be a crowd to welcome me? The Bangor Daily News article shared my Ellsworth arrival information in their story, so I didn't know what to expect. If there was ever a time for me to NOT miss a turn, it was now. But I did. I rode right past the turn into the Lodge. Scott made the turn and everyone else followed him as I kept rolling down Route 3 toward the town. I pulled off the side of the road and waited for an opening in the busy traffic to pull a U-turn. Cars kept coming from both directions. I could see back to the turnoff for the Lodge, which had a long lane in—the riders were waiting for me to turn around. Finally, I got my bike turned and headed back to the entrance of the Lodge. I pulled in and slowly rode past all the bikes. They filed in line behind me and we made our entrance. I pulled all the way through, stopping right in front of the TV news camera. There was a small crowd and some more bikers gathered there. They cheered as we rode in. I waved to everyone and the TV news reporter started her interview. That was followed by the newspaper reporter. Once I got the interviews out of the way, I could greet my supporters, some I knew, some I did not recognize. In the crowd was my friend Steve, who runs a motorcycle Facebook page. Steve had bought me my vanity license plate. My motorcycle mechanic, Stanley was there. I hugged him and told him the bike ran awesome the whole trip. I approached a woman I didn't recognize and introduced myself. It was one of those out of context moments. She was wearing sunglasses and warm jacket. It was Melanie, my oncology nurse. Oh my goodness, of course I knew her—she was an angel throughout all of my cancer care. Melanie was the reason I went ziplining at my first ovarian cancer retreat. I couldn't believe she had come out on a Saturday to welcome me home. My friend Michael Reisman from the Beth C. Wright Cancer Resource Center was there. Without Michael's help, I could never have managed the fundraising aspect of Teal on Wheels. It was so great to see so many familiar faces. An older couple approached me and I introduced myself. They introduced themselves as T, just T, and Helen. They shared a story about their daughter, who died in her

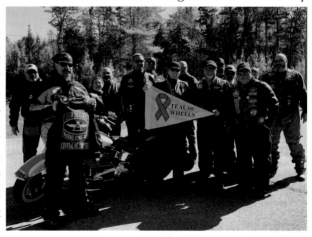

*The riders that escorted me home*

50s from ovarian cancer. Both T and Helen were wearing a teal ribbon cancer pin on their jackets. They told me that they read about my ride in the Bangor Daily News and wanted to come to meet me. I was so touched. Helen said, "You remind us of our daughter."

207

I couldn't think of any better way for me to complete my ride. My Widows Sons friends were heading out to lunch and invited us along. We were 25 miles from the ferry terminal and we just wanted to get home, so we declined their offer. We wanted to ride the very last leg alone, so we said our goodbyes and our thanks, saddled up, and rolled back out onto Route 3 heading east.

We made our way to the ferry and pulled in line. Waiting at the ferry terminal in Bass Harbor was my high school friend, Kreg, and his wife, Martha. They were on vacation in Acadia National Park and drove over to Bass Harbor to see me. So many people were going out of their way to welcome me home.

As we boarded the ferry for home, on this bright sunny afternoon, I was grateful—grateful for all the places I had vis-

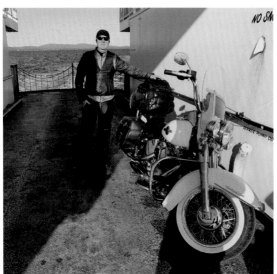

*On the ferry heading home*

ited and for all the people I had met along the way. I was grateful for all of my family and friends back home. I was grateful that I had made it home safely. I was grateful that I had succeeded in my mission of raising awareness about ovarian cancer by sharing my story and giving away 770 symptom cards to people I met on my journey. I had also succeeded in raising money that I would be able to donate to several ovarian cancer non-profits. Most of all, I was grateful for Charlie—who always supported me in everything I wanted to do. Now we were heading home to celebrate all that we had accomplished together.

I parked my bike on the deck of the ferry and climbed

up to the wheelhouse to see my friend, Captain Bob. Bob was on duty the day I left Swan's Island and it seemed fitting that he would be taking me home.

When the ferry docked on Swan's Island and we drove up the causeway, we were greeted by the same group of supporters that had bid me a fond farewell 40 days earlier. This time they were there to welcome me home. Brian and his wife, Kathy, had one of the island's firetrucks parked at the ferry terminal and were sitting in it with the siren blaring. After a quick stop to say hello and get some hugs from my wellwishers, Brian pulled out in front of Charlie and me and we followed the firetruck, with the siren blaring and the horn honking, all the way across the island to our home. On Swan's Island, a single firetruck with two motorcycles following constitutes a parade—and on that day, a welcome home parade.

We pulled the motorcycles into the boathouse where we store them. Before shutting off my bike, I checked my mileage one last time. I had ridden 6,198 miles across this great country—over 5,000 of those miles were solo. I had been away from home for 40 days. I had traveled through 19 different states and had visited 8 National Parks. My longest riding day was 306 miles. My shortest was 12 miles. I had overcome severe dehydration in the Smoky Mountains of Tennessee. I had overcome my fear and ridden across the Rocky Mountains. I had ridden in strong winds, oppressive heat, cold temperatures, torrential rain, lightning, and even hail. I had done it all and had arrived back home safely.

Once again, my heart was full of joy. How was I so lucky to have so many people that cared about me—what did I do to deserve such a great life? Some would say, how wonderful can a life be living with stage IV cancer? I'll admit, it is hard, but if you can find the courage to navigate your journey—you can have a beautiful life.

# AFTERWORD:
# ACHIEVING MY GOAL

I want to share a final story from my journey with you about a woman I have yet to meet. Her name is Mandi. We haven't been able to meet in person, even though she only lives about 50 miles from me. I only know her from her Facebook posts and through the private messages we exchange on Facebook Messenger, but I feel deeply connected to her. We've exchanged holiday greeting cards, and I even sent her a necklace in the mail a while back. I've met Mandi's husband, Brent, her sister-in-law, Tracie, and her brother-in-law, Howard, but I have yet to meet Mandi.

Who is she? And how are we connected? For me, Mandi represents everything that I set out to accomplish with Teal on Wheels. She first contacted me through Facebook Messenger, on October 17, 2019, two weeks after I returned from my cross country trip. This is part of the message that she sent to me:

*"I want to say thank you from the bottom of my heart. You shared your TEAL on WHEELS story with a local Shrine motorcycle chapter during their annual Tarbox Ride on June 2, 2019. My husband, Brent, is the Past Master of the Pleiades Lodge #173. You took the time to talk to him, tell him a bit of your story, and give him your card (one of my ovarian cancer symptom cards) an act that had such an impact that I can truly never thank you enough.*

*I've been sick with an unknown diagnosis for 2 years. I finally pushed for an appointment in August and got a referral to a Gynecologist. She assured me my pains were not gynecologic, but she ordered a trans vaginal ultrasound to appease my concerns. It came back positive for a mass. In the meantime I had a CT scan that showed no changes from 6 months ago with no pelvic mass. I was shocked and headed to Boston 2 days later on October 6. Needless to say, I was just discharged Tuesday, October 15, after a full hysterectomy and tumor removal. From here, we look into treatment options.*

*If you hadn't spoken with my husband, told him of the symptoms, I might never have pushed like I did. I'm so very thankful that you spoke with my husband. I feel like you saved my life and I cannot repay you. THANK YOU."*

When I finished reading Mandi's message, I cried. I wanted to meet her right away, but she was not finished with her cancer treatment. She would have to go through chemotherapy first, so I had to wait. Shortly after that, the Covid-19 pandemic struck and that delayed our meeting. We will meet at some point. I just don't know when.

Mandi's message was the proof I needed to know that I had made a difference. By sharing my story and handing out ovarian cancer symptom cards, I had achieved my goal of raising awareness about ovarian cancer. I never expected to hear back from anybody that I gave a card to. My hope is that at some point, maybe 5 years down the road, a woman that I met, who might develop the vague symptoms of ovarian cancer: *abdominal bloating, quickly feeling full when eating, change in bowel habits, frequent need to urinate, back or pelvic pain, and fatigue*—will know what to do. I hope that even if

she doesn't remember the specific symptoms, that she will remember meeting me because of the unique way I traveled. I
hope that she will remember my story about ovarian cancer, and
that she will look up the symptoms. My goal is to empower wom-
en everywhere to become better advocates for their own health
needs. Mandi's message, just weeks after returning home from
my trip, confirmed that what I had set out to do, I had accomplished. But my mission is not done—it's a long way from over. I
will continue to share my story and my ovarian cancer symptom
cards everywhere I go.

# Acknowledgments

First, I need to thank my husband, Charlie. I could not have started, let alone completed, TEAL on WHEELS, without his neverending support. As the idea turned into reality, Charlie helped me brainstorm ideas and overcome challenges. I would never have been able to ride the first mile, let alone 6,198 miles, without his support and encouragement.

The name for the trip, Teal on Wheels, was the idea of Margaret Mastrangelo. Margaret, an ovarian cancer survivor and good friend, was instrumental from day one in making my dream happen. She spent endless hours on the phone with me discussing all the details and working with me to make it all happen. Thank you, Margaret, for your friendship and your guidance.

Thank you to Sarah O'Neil, my health coach, for helping me find the courage to start writing when I needed a purpose.

This book would never have come to completion if it were not for my dear friend, Caroline Dane. Caroline had edited many things that I had written in the past, mostly short reports, but when I approached her about editing this book for me, she gladly accepted the challenge. Caroline read through my draft chapters, marking them up and quickly returning them, so I could continue writing. I wrote the book and completed the book design, from start to finish, in just over four months. Many people told me it couldn't be done in that time frame, but I like a good challenge. Caroline believed in me and encouraged me every step of the way.

I'd like to give a big shout out to my volunteer readers, who responded to my request to read a draft version of the book and provide feedback to me. They are Kate Tagai, Rob Pannier, and Margaret Mastrangelo. Their thoughtful comments and constructive criticism helped me to write a better book. Thank you all.

Thank you to Scott Harriman for proofreading the chapter called Brotherhood and making sure I got all the facts correct regarding the Masonic way of life.

I would like to thank Karen Pettit, owner of Highway 101 Harley-Davidson, for taking delivery of my motorcycle on the West Coast. The professionalism and kindness that she showed me was greatly appreciated. I felt confident knowing my bike was being delivered to her dealership. Thank you, Karen.

I would also like to thank everyone in the medical field that has provided care for me since my cancer journey began over five years ago. You have helped me surpass my original prognosis of five years. Thank you all for providing me with compassionate care every step of the way.

I want to thank all my family and friends for your support and love. You make my life better by being in it.

There are so many people to thank and I cannot possibly list them all. I want to thank the many generous donors who supported me and my cause. I wasn't sure I could reach my $50,000 fundraising goal, but people believed in me and supported me. In the end, the goal was not only reached, but exceeded.

I would like to acknowledge all the women who have received an ovarian cancer diagnosis, especially my Turning the Tide Sisters. Over the years, I have watched as many of you have struggled with your disease, some ultimately losing their lives. I honor each and every one of you. You have shown me how to live my life with courage. You are my true heroes.

Last, but certainly not least, thank you to Anne Tonachel for all that you do for women with ovarian cancer. I did not know that the day we met at Dana Farber in Boston would be a day that would change my life forever. Being part of the Turning the Tide Ovarian Cancer Retreat Sisterhood has meant so much to me. The love and kindness that you show to each one of the women who find their way to your retreat is remarkable. You are truly one of a kind, Anne.

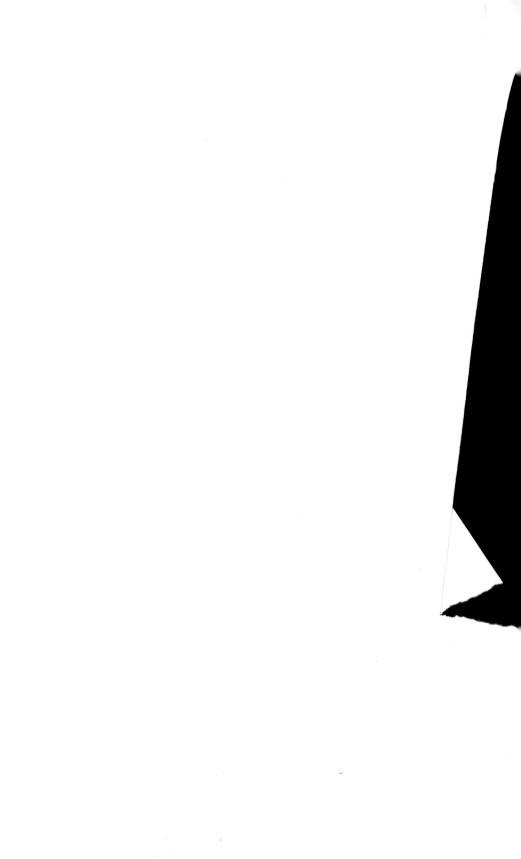

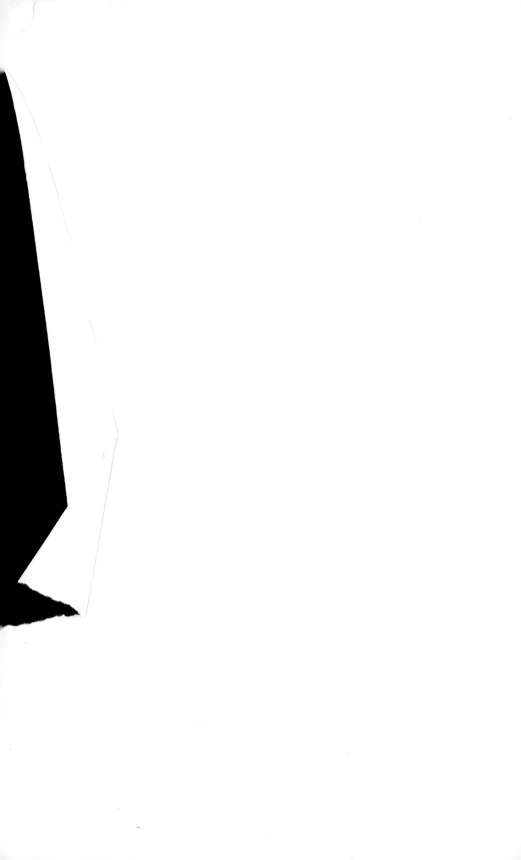

# Credits

**Cover design and book layout** - Donna Wiegle

**Photos:** All of the photos presented in this book are courtesy of the author, Donna Wiegle, except for the following:

Cover Photo - Charlie Wiegle

Page 30 - Eva Kasell

Page 64 - Karen Pettit

Page 72 - Al Hawes

Page 171 - Carolynn Loan

Page 185 - Donna Weisel

Page 193 - Ed Schwabe

Page 196 - Amy Kurman

**Fact checking:**
Page 51 - Three Great Principles of Freemasonry
(www.kingsolomonlodge54.com/3-principles-of-freemasonry)